ABANDONED PERRYSBURG

THE J. N. ADAM MEMORIAL HOSPITAL

BRIAN CRAY

AMERICA THROUGH TIME®
ADDING COLOR TO AMERICAN HISTORY

America Through Time is an imprint of Fonthill Media LLC
www.through-time.com
office@through-time.com

Published by Arcadia Publishing by arrangement with Fonthill Media LLC
For all general information, please contact Arcadia Publishing:
Telephone: 843-853-2070
Fax: 843-853-0044
E-mail: sales@arcadiapublishing.com
For customer service and orders:
Toll-Free 1-888-313-2665

www.arcadiapublishing.com

First published 2019

ISBN 978-1-63499-164-3

Typeset in Trade Gothic 10pt on 15pt
Printed and bound in England

CONTENTS

For my wife, Kelly Cray, and her aunt, Monique Landry.
Without your help and support this would have not been possible.

1

THE WHITE DEATH:
A Brief History on Tuberculosis and its Effects on Perrysburg, NY

The big city lights of industrialized America shine bright, boasting "must-have" products and services, but through time, often what thrived in the past now lays defunct in a field of overgrowth, with bits of rubble and the force of Mother Nature quickly creeping its fingertips up her empty walls. Whether in the city, its outskirts or in the rural countryside, these abandoned relics slowly waste away, becoming pieces of forgotten history. How does this happen? Myriad reasons affect their demise, most of which boils down to funding, changing of ownership or repurposing. In the case of the J. N. Adam Memorial Hospital in Perrysburg, NY, the inherent factor became a combination of the latter and ultimately, time! As such, operations ceased to exist as a tuberculosis sanitarium in the 1960s and again as a developmental center for the disabled in 1991, when she shut her doors for the last time.

Perrysburg, NY, is a small town located southeast of Lake Erie in Cattaraugus County. According to the 2010 census records, the town's population was 1,626 people. As of 2016, it decreased to an estimated 1,584 people, maintaining its steady decline since the 1970s.[1] On December 31, 2011, "Perrysburg," the census-designated place and former village, dissolved after voters approved 60-9 on March 16, 2011, in a referendum for its dissolution, which completed in 2011.[2]

Originally formed in 1814 and called the "Town of Perry," it was named after Commodore Oliver Hazard Perry.[3] In 1818, the town changed its name to "Perrysburgh" and eventually the spelling changed to "Perrysburg."[4] The town covers a distance of 28.5 square miles according to the United States Census Bureau.[5] Due to its proximity to the Great Lakes, it experiences lake-effect snow and rainfall resulting in heavy precipitation. Some have referred to it as the snow capital of Western New York, but beneath that ivory blanket is much more than just a small town. There is much rich history trapped among those enchanted hills where she claws away at her crumbling walls from the harsh elements of time as her memories slowly fade away brick-by-brick to pages of a book. This is her history; the history of the J. N. Adam Memorial Hospital. This is how she once thrived as one of the leading institutes of heliotherapy in New York State, researching light as an application for medicine.

Tuberculosis is an airborne pathogen caused by Mycobacterium tuberculosis, which are rod-shaped bacterium that affect the lungs, bones, joints, genitals or nervous system depending on whether the individual exhibits pulmonary or extrapulmonary tuberculosis.[6] Robert Koch, a German microbiologist and physician, became the first person to successfully identify the bacteria responsible for tuberculosis on March 24, 1882. This day is now designated as World TB Day.[7] Commonly referred to as Consumption or "The White Plague," this infectious disease killed one out of every seven people in Europe and the United States in the late 1800s.[8] TB still continues to plague us today, despite an antibiotic cure that has existed since the 1940s.[9] According to a 1928 edition of *Grit-Grin,* "The lowest death rate for the disease ever recorded in the state of New York was 89.1 deaths per 100,000 populations in 1926." Despite one-third of the world's population today carrying Mycobacterium tuberculosis, only about 10 percent of those individuals suffer from the disease in their lifetimes while the rest live in remission.[10]

By the 1900s, 40 percent of Americans resided in cities as the industrial revolution caused a shift in populations, and with it, brought much change in the production and distribution of food.[11] Obesity ground its roots like stone between 1870 and 1914 due to these industrialized food methods of mass production.[12] City life also triggered the onslaught of concern for food safety, quality control, clean water and sanitation practices. These factors all ultimately contributed to the epidemics of scarlet fever, typhoid, cholera and tuberculosis.

Nowadays, we take all of these for granted, but in the early 1900s, they tremendously affected the quality of life, especially in cities where crowded and unsanitary living conditions became a Petri dish of contagious disease festering among the filthy streets. With improper hygiene bolstering disease, a raise for concern spiked amongst cities, and preventative methods ensued to hinder the spread of such crippling plagues. In 1896, the "No Spitting" legislation passed.[13] Citations and punishments as hefty as jail time resulted to ward off the spread of tuberculosis. Then in 1904, Edward Livingston Trudeau founded the National Association for the Study and Prevention of Tuberculosis, which is now the American Lung Association.[14]

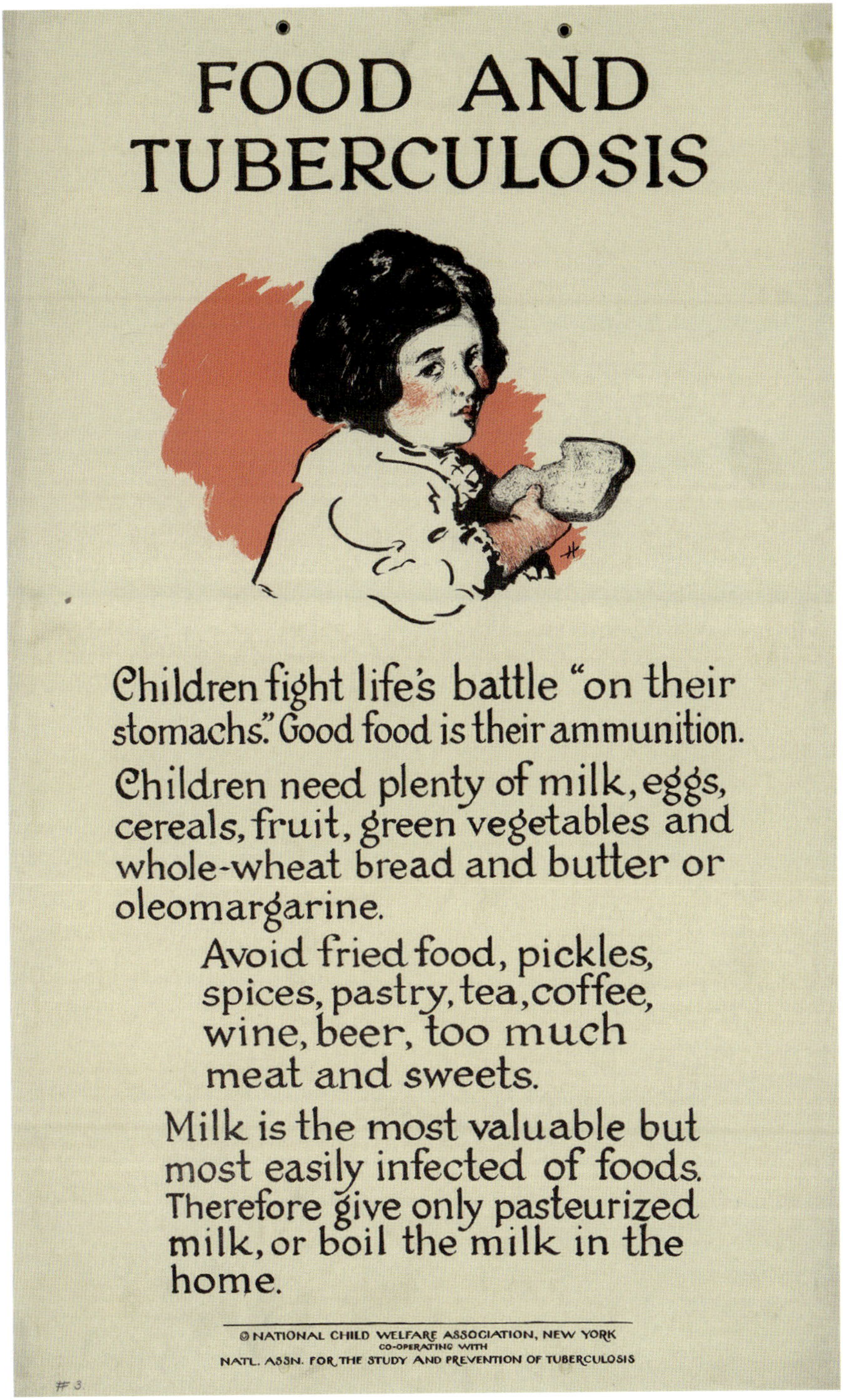
FOOD AND TUBERCULOSIS
Children fight life's battle "on their stomachs." Good food is their ammunition.
Children need plenty of milk, eggs, cereals, fruit, green vegetables and whole-wheat bread and butter or oleomargarine.
Avoid fried food, pickles, spices, pastry, tea, coffee, wine, beer, too much meat and sweets.
Milk is the most valuable but most easily infected of foods. Therefore give only pasteurized milk, or boil the milk in the home.
© NATIONAL CHILD WELFARE ASSOCIATION, NEW YORK
CO-OPERATING WITH
NATL. ASSN. FOR THE STUDY AND PREVENTION OF TUBERCULOSIS

[Photo by National Child Welfare Association]

In 1905, he founded the American Sanitarium Society, which is now the American Thoracic Society.[15] Both groups continue to research and fight pulmonary diseases hoping to eradicate TB by the year 2050, but it was not until 1944, when Doctor Selman Waksman of Rutgers University in NJ discovered streptomycin, a new drug that completely eradicated the bacterium causing tuberculosis.[16, 17]

The years between the fight for a cure mark a fledgling age of due learning and increased regulations followed. Pasteurization laws helped prevent the contamination of milk. Prior to this, bone tuberculosis was contributed to the infected milk from cows afflicted with tuberculin that passed it on to consumers, and in such cases, the drinking of said milk was crippling.[18] Contaminated food in the early 1900s also sparked controversies and on June 30, 1906, President Theodore Roosevelt signed the Pure Food and Drug Act along with the Meat Inspection Act.[19] While there is minimal chance of contracting TB through eating infected bovine TB cows, these acts ensured that livestock met sanitary standards, mandating that the U.S. Department of Agriculture (USDA) examine all cattle before and after slaughtering and processing them for public consumption.[20]

Statistical data from 1907 shows that tuberculosis killed 198.5 people per 100,000 populations in New York State with 76,650 deaths from tuberculosis in the United States that year.[21] These rates fluctuated up and down. By 1908, "The White Plague" grabbed the attention of the world from September 25th to October 12th where a meeting of the International Congress on Tuberculosis took place in Washington D.C. displaying charts, diagrams and statistical data on the death toll surrounding the deadly contagion.[22]

Tuberculosis and other epidemics continued to spread like wildfire as the city frequented contaminated water sources. Before indoor plumbing, outhouses were often shared with anyone of the hundred people living in a tenement. These holes in the ground festered with feces, vermin and disease, which seeped into local waterways contaminating drinking water.

It was not until 1935 that New York State Health Department founded the Buffalo Sewer Authority in an effort to stop polluting the Niagara River, which bred copious communicable diseases.[23] This authority created a sewage system that directed all sewers to a treatment facility on Bird Island to eliminate solid waste and to chlorinate recyclable drinking water for the public.[24]

According to *Tuberculosis Transmission by Waste Waters: A Review* from 1957, many studies around the world identified active virulent tubercle bacilli from discharged sewage near tuberculosis sanitaria along with dairy and slaughterhouses with infected cattle. Theories postulating the spread of tuberculosis through contaminated water, contaminated vegetables irrigated by said water and drinking

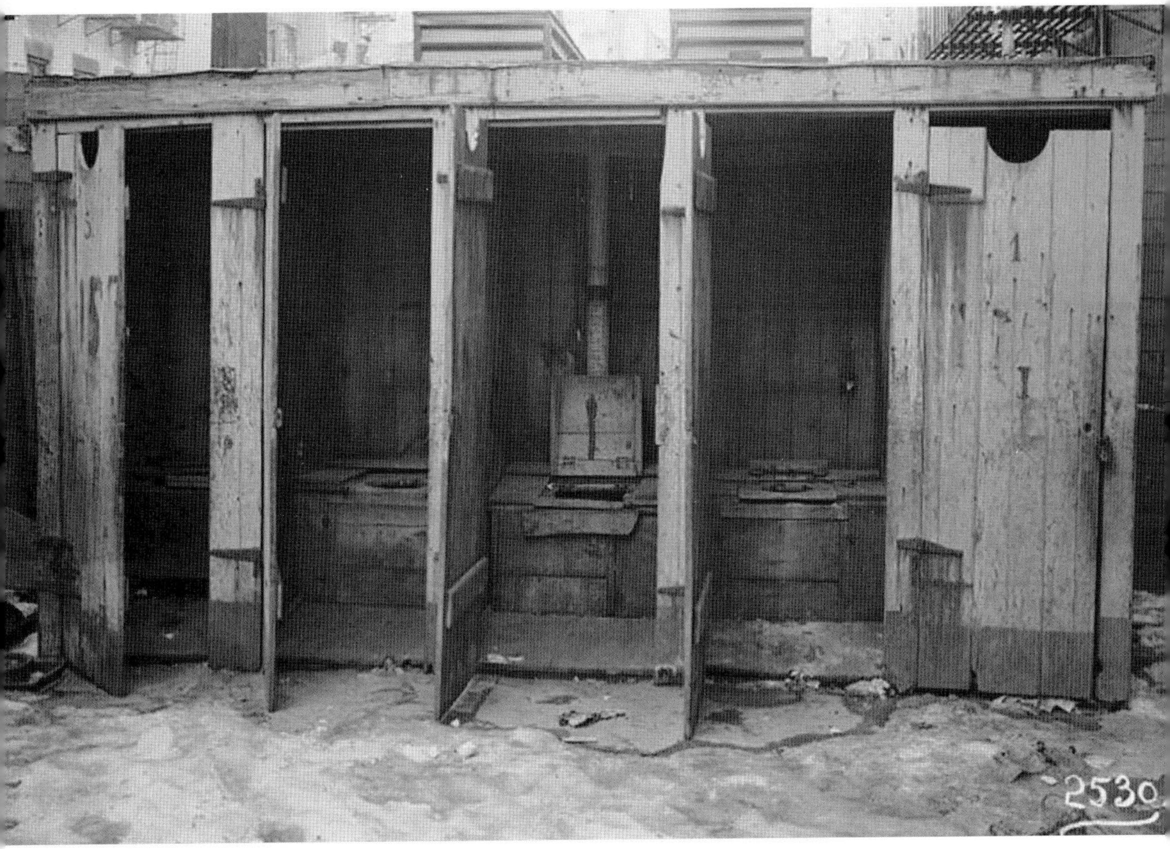

Here is a row of outhouses in New York City. [Photo by Irma and Paul Milstein from The New York Public Library Digital Collections]

contaminated milk drew similar conclusions in regards to conventional sewage treatments. Scientists suggested a combination of current sewage treatments in addition to the purification and chlorination of sewage to disinfect active virulent tubercle bacilli. Studies by Schalk found that contaminated barns in North Dakota with active tubercle bacilli survived up to twelve months, even through the harshest of winters. Musehold, Sollazo, Jusatz, and Kraus all recommended induction of well-oxidized effluent chlorination to disinfect contaminated sewage resulting from the fececs and sputum of tuberculosis sanitaria, slaughterhouses and dairy operations. The risk of contracting tuberculosis from contaminated sputum and sewage shows minimal support, except in cases involving swimming and near drowning in polluted waters, with cases as early as 1947 from Gaustad. However, these eerie public health and sanitation standards definitely spurred a cause for concern for wastewater treatment in the prevention and spread of communicable diseases.[25]

There was a steady decline of tuberculosis at the turn of the twentieth century in New York. Living standards, improvements on public health, the eradication of bovine TB, improved logging efforts of TB and the expansion of educational awareness all contributed to a decline in mortality rates from the disease.[26] If you refer to Figure 1 of *Trends in Mortality of Tuberculosis Patients in the United States: The Long-term Perspective*, you can see a continued decline in mortality rates associated from tuberculosis and as anti-tuberculosis drugs hit the market in the 1940s, there is a further decline.

As mortality rates declined throughout the twentieth century, with a plateau in the 1980s, and a steady decrease into the twenty-first century, the use for heliotherapy facilities became defunct and ceased to exist. Despite efforts to find more effective vaccinations for tuberculosis, currently only Bacille Calmette-Guerin (BCG) exists, and is not widely utilized for immunization in small children in the United States, according to the Centers for Disease Control and Prevention.[27] Cases of TB still very much exist throughout the United States among other first-world countries of today, but are more prevalent in third-world countries like Africa and parts of Southeast Asia. As the world waged battle against tuberculosis in the early 1900s, a few men innovated alternative methods against surgical and pulmonary tuberculosis through the means of heliotherapy, one of which was its creator, Dr. Rollier of Leysin, Switzerland.

2

DR. ROLLIER'S METHOD OF HELIOTHERAPY:

A Brief History on the First Sun Cure Clinic

J. N. Adam Memorial Hospital in Perrysburg, NY, first introduced Dr. Rollier's method of heliotherapy into the United States of America in 1913.[1] Dr. Rollier became an advocate of heliotherapy after working under his mentor, Professor Kocher. He noticed the unsatisfactory results attributed to operating on bone and joint tuberculosis despite Kocher's knowledge and credentials.[2] Treating the disease strictly as a surgical one allowed Rollier to explore other ideologies by Finsen who discovered the effectiveness of sunlight against tuberculosis.[3] The outdoors, fresh air and high altitudes all contributed to the improvements of tuberculosis, and in 1903, Rollier opened the first heliotherapy sanitarium in Leysin, Switzerland, tackling the contagion through the application of light.[4] Like every operation, his efforts started off very small, attending to a few patients, but quickly escalated to 1,000 patients.

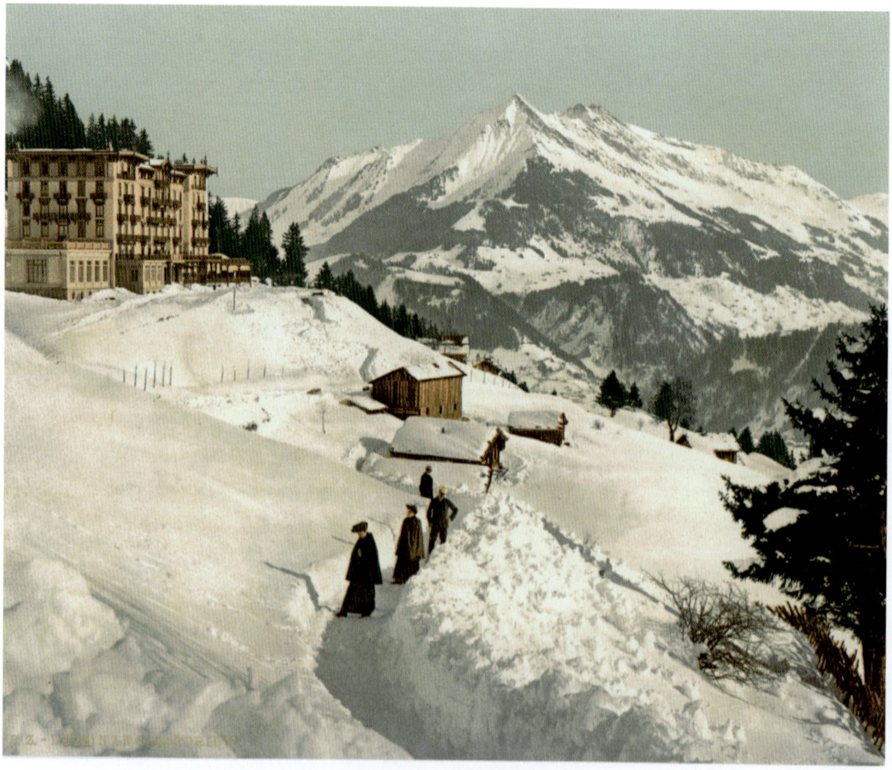

This is the sanatorium in Leysin, Switzerland circa 1890. [Photo retrieved from the Library of Congress]

Dr. Rollier was one of the first physicians to meticulously administer heliotherapy as a systematic treatment to mitigate the pain of crippled and emaciated tuberculin infected individuals solely using ultraviolet light. He believed the sun affected the skin in three ways through "latent hyperemia, pigmentation and thickening of the epidermis."[5] Rollier was not the first person to extensively foster the healing properties of sunlight. Many others administered the sun cure as early as 1889; however, his research and statistical records over ten years of practicing heliotherapy became the first of its kind for the medical world.[6] They started recognizing heliotherapy as a rational treatment for TB when he published a report in 1913 detailing his studies on its application upon tuberculin patients. As a result of the 1,129 cases he treated, more than 1,000 patients were cured of tuberculosis.[7, 8]

Dr. Rollier developed specific guidelines and routines for his patients undergoing heliotherapy. He made these methods available for other physicians to adopt at other sanitaria to work in the fight against the number one contagion plaguing the world. Through administering his definitive approach of heliotherapy, patients gradually acclimated to the outdoors, adjusting to the elements of Mother Nature in a healthy and steady manner. This meant no solar exposure took place during their first three to ten days of entry into the program, but instead, the patient adjusted slowly to the outdoors by sleeping inside the sanitarium with the doors or windows open at first. Then a physician wheeled the patient out to the open veranda on a bed and slowly acclimated to the outdoors over the next days until he spent much of the whole day outside. During this period, the physician administered samples of a patient's temperature, pulse, blood and urine, and using subjective intellect, gradually recommended a dosage of solar exposure, which was performed on a bed, a couch or the floor.[9] It was important that the sun cure be administered at least one hour after eating and no sooner than a half hour before a meal. Below is an outline of Dr. Rollier's method of heliotherapy.[10]

DAY 1 – Patients typically wear head protection in the form of a linen cap, a sun bonnet or lay under a bed awning. Sun glasses are worn to protect patients' eyes. Pajamas or nightgowns are also worn as patients acclimate to sun exposure treatments. If necessary, depending on the time of year and weather, a five-foot movable screen is used to prevent crosswinds and to protect patients from breeze. Chilling could result in dangerously detrimental side-effects like pneumonia. As such, if it is summertime, do not administer sun cure during the hottest points of the day. Instead, use the morning and late afternoons to avoid nausea, vomiting, headache and fever. The feet experience a maximum of "four insolations" in five minute intervals per hour disregarding any lesions. Then using gauze or a wire screen cover the lesions until the whole body steadily acclimates to solar radiation over the coming days.[11]

DAY 2 – The feet experience a ten minute exposure while the legs experience a five minute exposure with the body covered from the knees to the head. This is done four times per hour with patients rotating from back to chest and vice versa.

DAY 3 – The feet experience a fifteen minute exposure, the legs experience a ten minute exposure, and the thighs experience a five minute exposure for a maximum of four times per hour.

DAY 4 – The feet experience full sunlight in hour intervals, the legs experience fifteen minute exposure, the thighs experience ten minute exposure, and the abdomen experiences five minute exposure a maximum of four times per hour.

DAY 5 - The feet and legs experience full sunlight in hour intervals, the thighs experience fifteen minute exposure, the abdomen experiences ten minute exposure, and the chest and back experience five minute exposures a maximum of four times per hour.

DAY 6 – The feet, legs and thighs experience full sunlight in hour intervals, the abdomen experiences fifteen minute exposure, and the chest and back experience ten minute exposures a maximum of four times per hour.[12]

All exposures are done anteriorly and posteriorly, switching positions each period of exposure until three to four hours of sun cure is achieved. Upon the completion of these preliminary treatments, the sinuses and lesions should receive exposure where only a loin cloth is employed to cover the appendage with a wire screen to defend against any flies.[13]

It is during this period that the patients are massaged with oil between each sun bath.[14] Once a chocolate-bronze pigmentation is achieved on the skin, the patient is said to gain a "resistance to germs." After just a few months of the sunshine prescription, the patient is rid of pain with a reduction in lesions and pus discharge, noticeable throughout the body. The thicker the pigmentation, the deeper the ultra violet rays penetrate the skin, which supposedly allowed children to run around in the snow without catching colds.[15]

Three to four hours of sun cure per day left copious time for boredom to ruminate throughout the rest of the day. So what did patients do? On top of sun baths, physicians administered air baths for approximately ten to twenty minutes.[16] When patients were not undergoing treatments, depending on the severity of their case, they either spent their days bed-ridden listening to earphones of radio concerts, while motion pictures, musicals or theatricals occupied the more active crowd.[17] According to Charles Stewart, who worked at the sanitarium as an x-ray technician, "shows with Marilyn Monroe, Danny Thomas and other performers came out once a year."[18]

The older patients occupied their time by working on the magazine *Grit-Grin*, which the sanitarium published on a monthly basis. A yearly subscription cost just a dollar while individual copies cost ten cents. Mr. Edmond Sendker worked in the General Factory Accountant Department at that time and he slowly handled any of the subscriptions related to the magazine. *Grit-Grin* was strictly a non-profit magazine whose sole purpose was to boost spirits of in-patients, as well as spread knowledge on the severity of tuberculosis, and how to treat it using Dr. Rollier's method of heliotherapy. *Grit-Grin* attained much of its support like other sanitaria publications of that time through mailing lists, advertising and subscriptions. The first publication was printed on January 1, 1914.[19, 20]

Depending on the weather, children frolicked among the woods and haystacks in the summertime, climbing trees and playing under the radiant sun, but never during the hottest point of the day. While in winter, with only a loin cloth covering there appendages, they skied down the rolling snowy hillsides, tobogganed, and played in the snow, under supervision of course, as not to catch a deathly chill adversely impacting their health.[21]

Aside from the normal activities of playing outside, J. N. Adam Memorial Hospital was the only hospital in the world to have a zoo for its patients.[22] Animals attributed happiness for patients of all kind, giving unconditional love, when all hope sequestered to turbid weather and its malignance.

With acres and acres of land, the hospital produced its own food. Vegetable gardens and fodder accompanied 250 acres and chicken houses and stables accompanied another 250 acres.[23] The farm consisted of a hen house with 1,500 White Leg-Horn Hens, which was where they acquired their fresh eggs.[24] Fresh milk came from their prized Holstein cows from which they had seventy-six, along with 100 hogs.[25] The farm also allotted space for a state-of-the-art horse barn and a cow barn featuring multiple grain silos.[26]

A combination of the sun cure, and a family atmosphere that promoted high spirits through entertainment, among the stunning views produced by this castle-like complex, all contributed to the support and application of Rollier's method of heliotherapy. Dr. Bendes, Dr. LoGrasso and Dr. Hyde's countless publications promoting the application of light for pulmonary and extrapulmonary cases of tuberculosis make it the first of its kind in the United States of America. Shortly after, other sanitaria followed in the footsteps of the J. N. Adam Memorial Hospital fostering its principles as the main treatment for tuberculosis before streptomycin surfaced in the 1940s and pasteurization laws reduced the spread of the disease from bovine infected cows.

The hospital implored for the image of a family atmosphere to outsiders, but its self-sustained environment, natural cure-all methods, self-published magazine, its dairy, vegetables, and maple syrup only masked the malevolence hiding its true skin behind a façade. After reading a firsthand account from Char Szabo-Perricelli's book *Her Inside Voice,* and also speaking with the town historian Jody Shaw, I confirmed some of my own suspicions about the "altruistic" intentions of the hospital.[27] In my opinion, they strictly existed for the sole purpose of glorifying research about heliotherapy.[28] Patient abuse and neglect may have surfaced as a result of torpid personnel and understaffing in the wards with only two to three nurses on duty for the upwards of forty rascals.[29,30] Nurses often strapped children into their beds to prevent them from wandering off at night and getting into mischief. They also stepped on bare toes of children who ran around the wards so they didn't have to chase after them again.

The story Szabo-Perricelli tells depicts the pain and suffering of young children who needed to cope with mental anguish and emotional abuse. They did so without the loving endearment of their parents as visitation was limited and often interfered with work schedules. It almost feels like a faceless mosaic of children and staff lurked the grounds like lifeless ghouls, and patients only knew their beds, for play time and friendships was a conjuring of the papers.[31]

But, some staff and patients disagree. Bias associated from one individual to another will always be a bi-polar expression of interpretations. Many "apparently recovered or arrested" cases often times ended with patients coming back to the facility to work as staff.[32, 33]

> "Camaraderie and comfortable social interaction existed" and "when patients were discharged, pots and pans shot off like fireworks while the car horn beeped," according to I.K., a former patient and employee of the sanitarium.[34, 35]

According to Dr. Mark Caldwell, author of *The Last Crusade: The War on Consumption 1862-1954,*

> many patients at sanitariums similar to the first tuberculosis sanitarium at Saranac Lake, operated by Dr. Trudeau, felt obligated to transcribe fake memoirs of cheerful experiences.[36]

So, it is not an impractical assumption to adapt Dr. Caldwell's statement to other sanitariums of that time period like the J. N. Adam Memorial Hospital, for instance.[37]

J. N. ADAM MEMORIAL HOSPITAL IN 1920

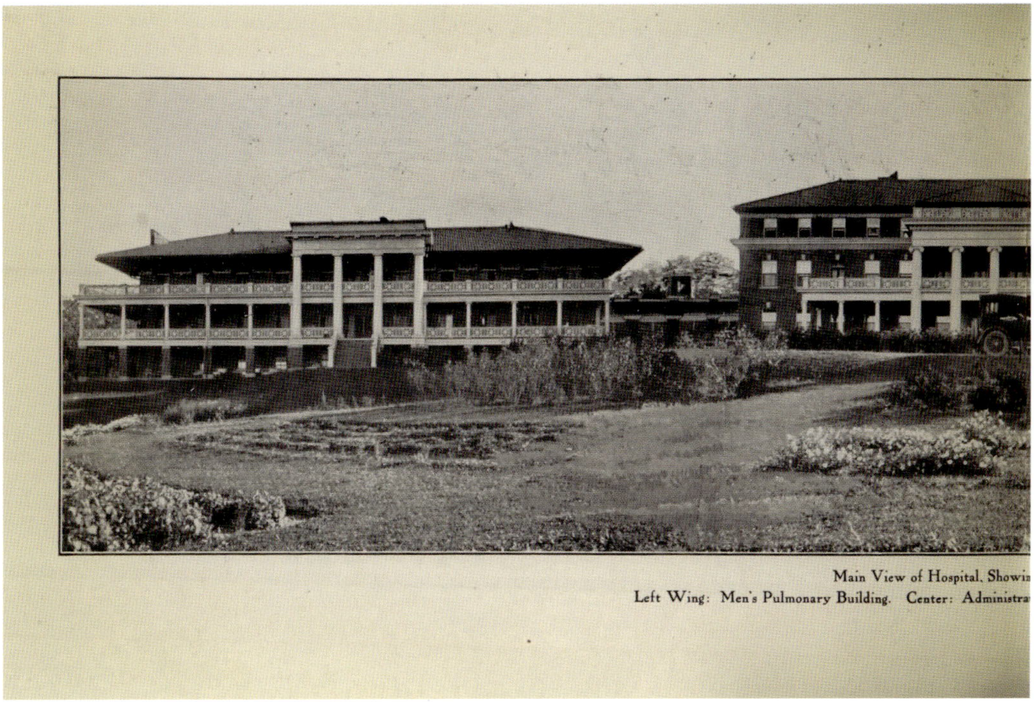

This is the J. N. Adam Memorial Hospital in her heyday. *[Photo by Frank Ruslander, 1920]*

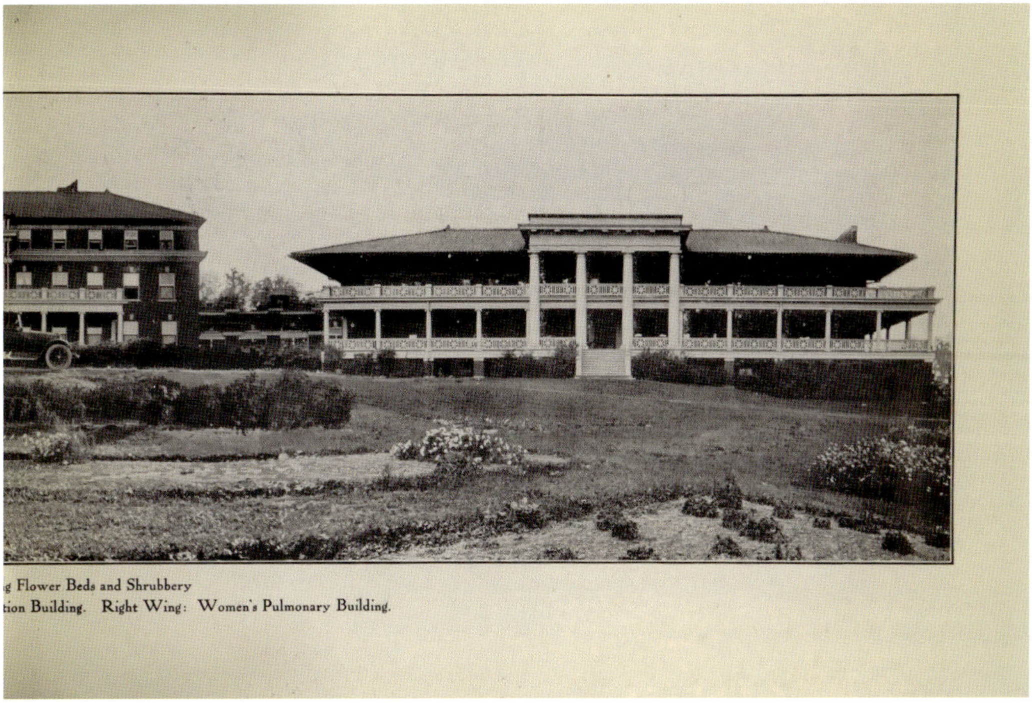

Back in 1920 she acted as a tuberculosis sanitarium treating hundreds of patients. *[Photo by Frank Ruslander, 1920]*

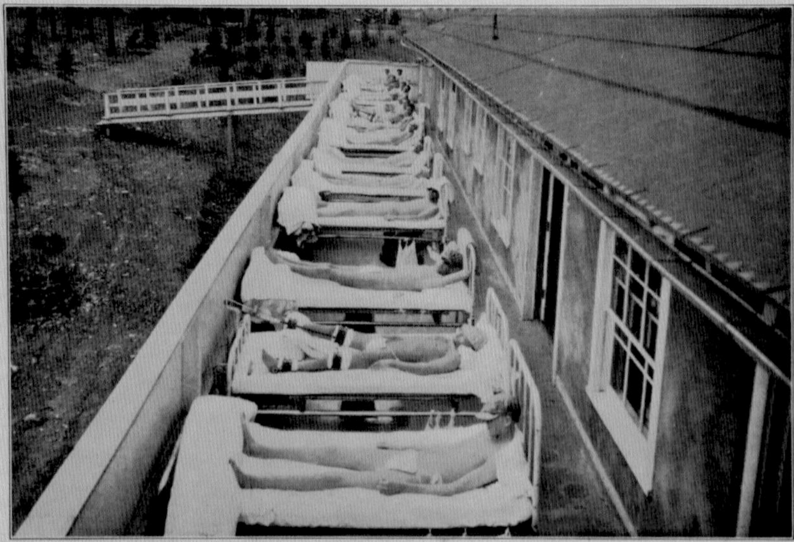

Surgical Cases taking Sun Cure
The Patients take Sun on their Entire Body from 3 to 4 Hours a Day

Every patient wears only a loin cloth to cover their appendages while they bask in the sun cure to ease their minds from terminal illness. *[Photo by Frank Ruslander, 1920]*

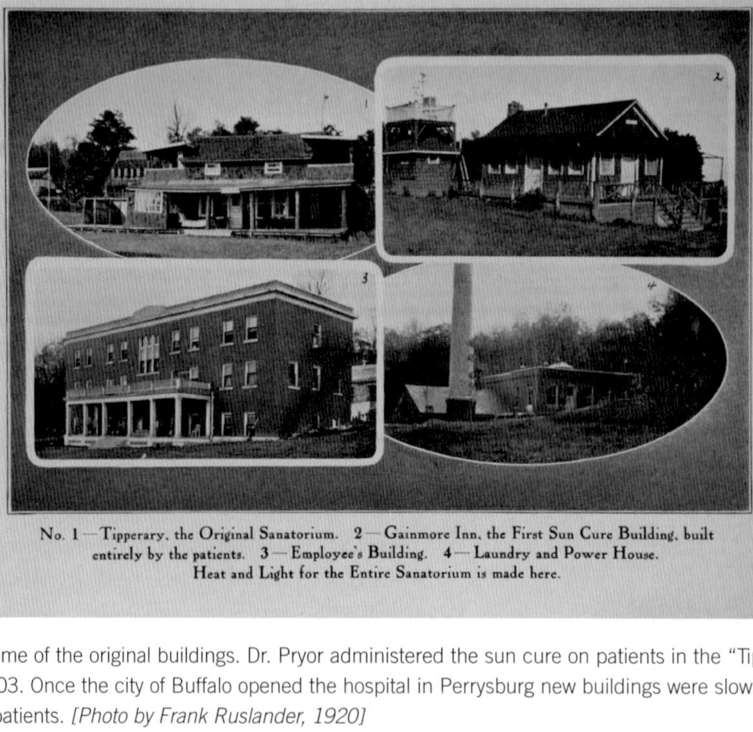

No. 1—Tipperary, the Original Sanatorium. 2—Gainmore Inn, the First Sun Cure Building, built entirely by the patients. 3—Employee's Building. 4—Laundry and Power House. Heat and Light for the Entire Sanatorium is made here.

These were some of the original buildings. Dr. Pryor administered the sun cure on patients in the "Tipperary" as early as 1903. Once the city of Buffalo opened the hospital in Perrysburg new buildings were slowly added to treat more patients. *[Photo by Frank Ruslander, 1920]*

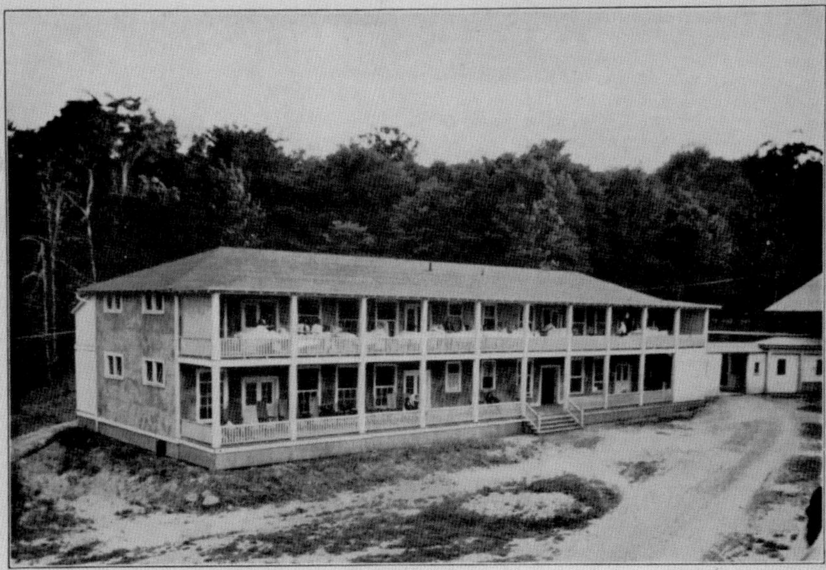

Men's Sun Cure Building
This Building Houses 50 Surgical Patients

[Photo by Frank Ruslander, 1920]

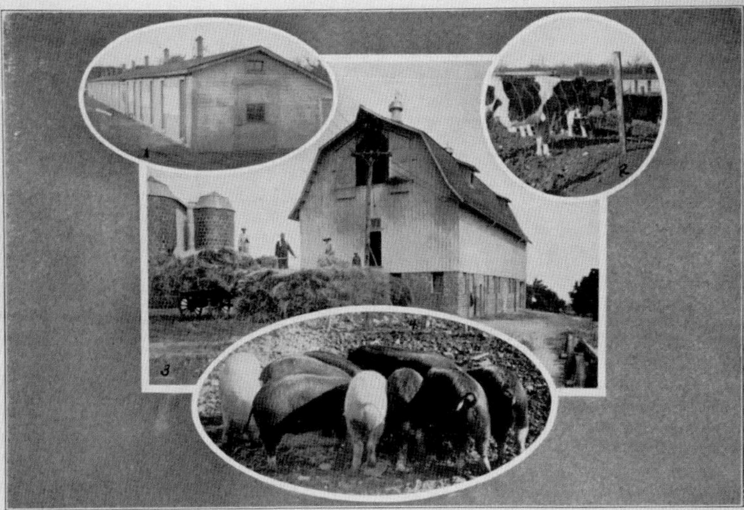

Our Modern Farm

No. 1. The Hen House; The Hospital Farm has 1500 White Leg-Horn Hens from which we get our fresh Eggs.
No. 2. Fresh Milk for the Patients is obtained from 76 Prize Holsteins.
No. 3. The up-to-date Horse Barn is shown here. A Cow Barn with Silos is shown at the Left.
No. 4. A few Prize Porkers. The Farm has 100 Hogs.

According to Fitzgerald, the sanitarium used 500 acres for producing her own food and tending livestock on the modern farm. *[Photo by Frank Ruslander, 1920]*

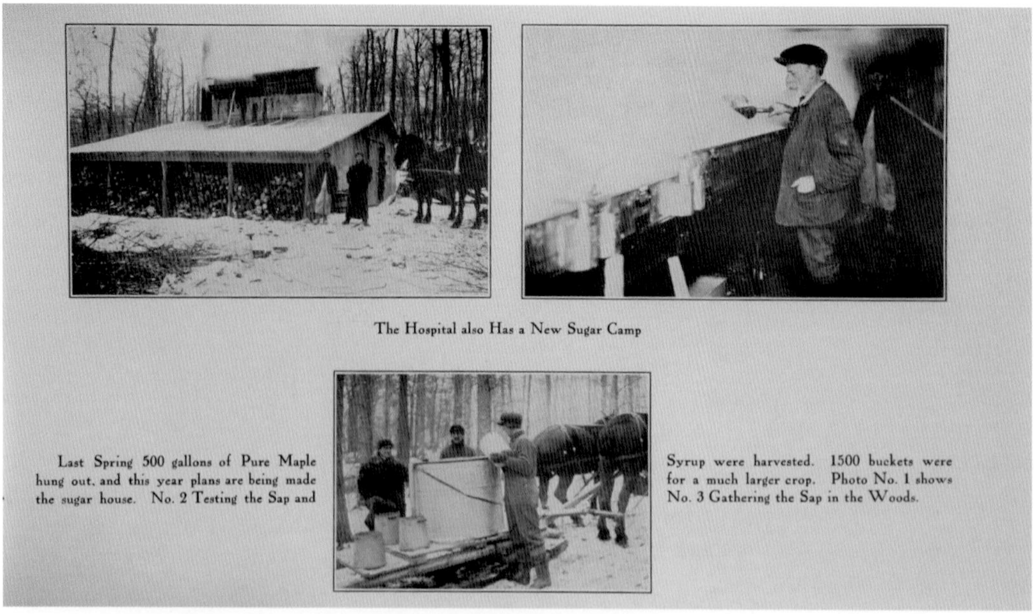
The Hospital also Has a New Sugar Camp

Last Spring 500 gallons of Pure Maple Syrup were harvested. 1500 buckets were hung out, and this year plans are being made for a much larger crop. Photo No. 1 shows the sugar house. No. 2 Testing the Sap and No. 3 Gathering the Sap in the Woods.

Vegetables, meats, eggs, milk and pork were not the only sustainable foods produced at the sanitarium. Maple syrup was also harvested as seen above. *[Photo by Frank Ruslander, 1920]*

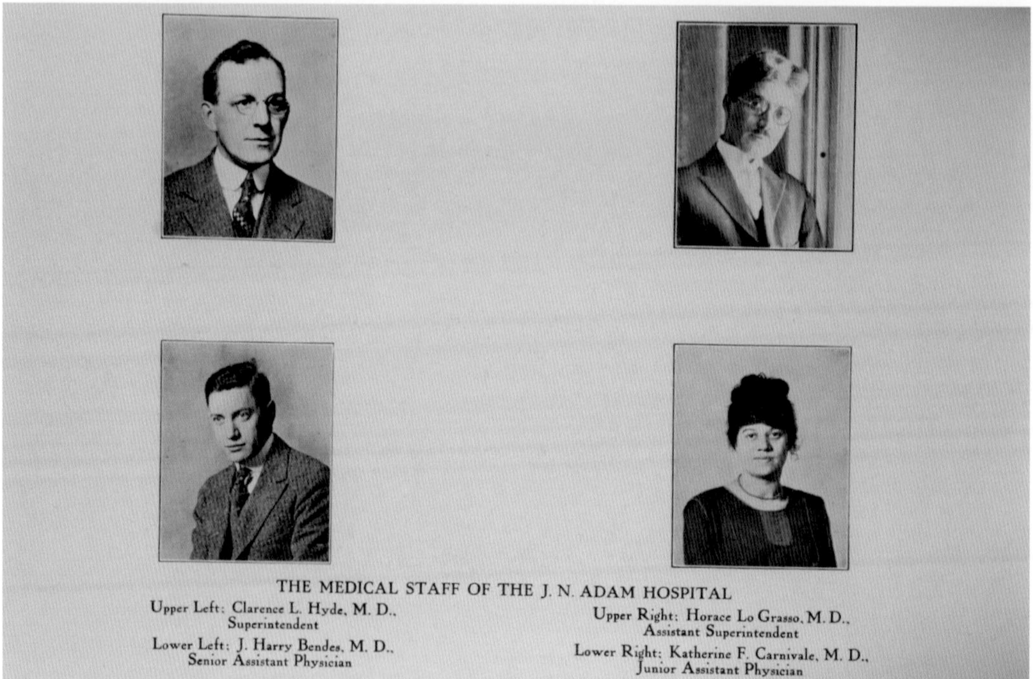
THE MEDICAL STAFF OF THE J. N. ADAM HOSPITAL

Upper Left: Clarence L. Hyde, M. D.,
Superintendent

Lower Left: J. Harry Bendes, M. D.,
Senior Assistant Physician

Upper Right: Horace Lo Grasso, M. D.,
Assistant Superintendent

Lower Right: Katherine F. Carnivale, M. D.,
Junior Assistant Physician

Hyde worked at the sanitarium until 1921. His successor, LoGrasso, worked at the hospital until retirement (Dalkowski, 2017; Szabo-Perricelli, 2016). Bendes moved on to Glen Lake Sanatorium in Oak Terrace, Minnesota, where he became an assistant medical director (Bendes, 1922). Carnivale worked at the sanitarium from 1918 to 1920. She moved on to diagnostic work examining thousands of chest x-rays in her career (*Supreme Court Appellate Division-Fourth Department,* 1940). *[Photo by Frank Ruslander, 1920]*

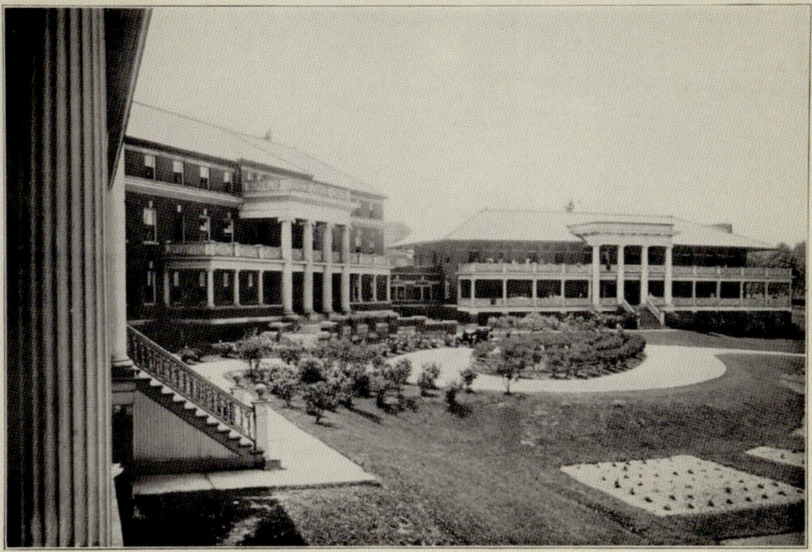

Front View of Main Building taken from Men's Pulmonary Pavilion

[Photo by Frank Ruslander, 1920]

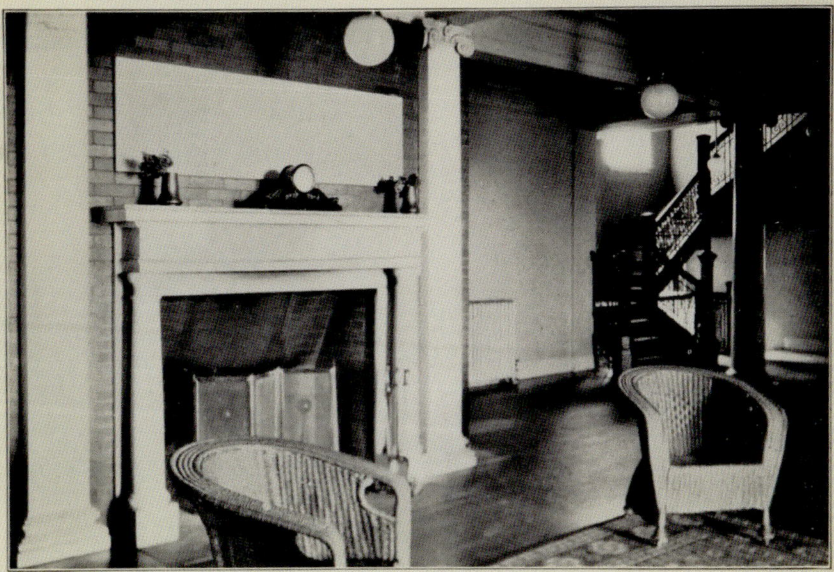

Main Entrance to Administration Building

This is inside the main entrance to the administration building when the floors still glistened with shiny wood, the walls shimmered with fresh paint, and the thought of decay never crossed a single mind (Frank Ruslander, 1920). *[Photo by Frank Ruslander, 1920]*

3

THE J. N. ADAM MEMORIAL HOSPITAL:

A Brief History on One of the First Heliotherapy Sanitariums in New York State

James Noble Adam climbed the ladder to fortune from hard work and determination. Originally a poor plebian and an errand boy from Scotland who made no more than a measly $1-a-week, he came to America and dabbled in a dozen years of politics, and thrived as a business owner for the largest store in Buffalo, NY, boosting his riches to $2,000,000.[1] What made him noble was not his last name, nor his wealth, but his philanthropy.

Back in the early 1900s, with the rise of tuberculosis and inadequate city and county hospitals unfit to properly administer therapies for afflicted citizens, Mayor James Noble Adam addressed this urgent malady arising in Buffalo, NY.[2] In the spring of 1909, with the help of the Hospital Commission of Buffalo, Dr. John H. Pryor and Mayor James Noble Adam introduced a bill to the legislature to design, build, outfit and operate a municipal hospital in New York State for the treatment of incipient and subclinical tuberculosis.[3] On March 25, 1909, the bill passed by the state legislature. With the "White Plague" running wild, the mayor hired John Hopper Coxhead to design the Buffalo Municipal Hospital for Incipient Tuberculosis (J. N. Adam Memorial Hospital), which Coxhead designed free of charge.[4] The mayor purchased the 293-acre parcel from his own personal fortune and donated it to the city. Subsequently, on December 18, 1909, the Buffalo City Council chose construction for the J. N. Adam Memorial Hospital, birthing her along the Cattaraugus Hills in Perrysburg, some 1,600 feet above sea level and becoming a superlative successor to Dr. Rollier's method of heliotherapy.[5]

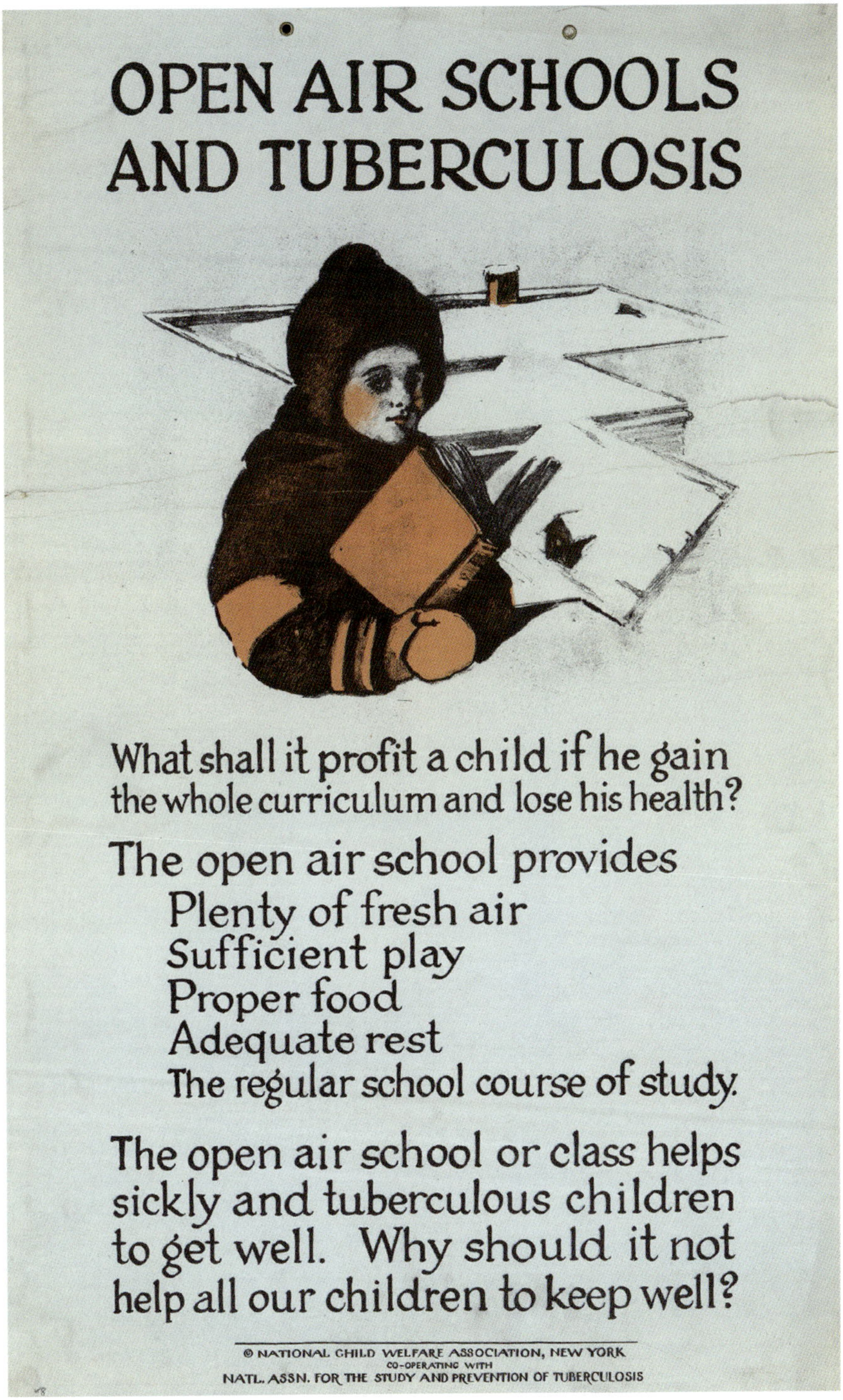
OPEN AIR SCHOOLS
AND TUBERCULOSIS
What shall it profit a child if he gain
the whole curriculum and lose his health?
The open air school provides
Plenty of fresh air
Sufficient play
Proper food
Adequate rest
The regular school course of study.
The open air school or class helps
sickly and tuberculous children
to get well. Why should it not
help all our children to keep well?
© NATIONAL CHILD WELFARE ASSOCIATION, NEW YORK
CO-OPERATING WITH
NATL. ASSN. FOR THE STUDY AND PREVENTION OF TUBERCULOSIS

[Photo by National Child Welfare Association]

On October 13, 1910, a contract of $160,000 was issued for any initial building costs, and upon completion, total costs slightly exceeded the upwards of $300,000.[6] The J. N. Adam Memorial Hospital completed construction on September 13, 1912, carried out by Charles Hager, with a formal opening on November 12, 1912, after almost three years of construction.[7] The hospital first consisted of only one small building, influenced by English architecture, the "Tipperary," which residents had not minded, as Dr. Pryor administered the sun cure to patients on a small scale as early as 1903, with the first patient being Bula M. Lincoln.[8] However, the community really did not want a colossal sanitarium in their town for fear of spreading disease.[9] Gradually, as the hospital became more established, and the community maintained its health, people became more accepting. Property values rose and the small little town of Perrysburg adjusted to the aiding therapeutic practices of heliotherapy, deeming the hospital a healing ground for those suffering and in need of treatments. The stigma changed and people embraced its altruism instead of treating it like an omen.

The idea behind the complex focused on nature to heal one's wounds and centralized its practices from Dr. Rollier's method of heliotherapy. The complex, situated on a sloping hilltop, deemed the splendid views of the open countryside along with the fresh flow of air and sun to cure tuberculosis. Patients basked among the loggias in the fresh air practicing the "sunshine cure," a natural healing method of Swiss origin.

At first, the facility catered to a capacity of 128 in-patients, accompanied by three nurses and two physicians.[10] The sanitarium utilized two wings and an administration building, but over the years added additions, and increased its capacity to 420 in-patients. In total, the J. N. Adam Memorial Hospital comprised of fifty-seven buildings.[11] The edifices on the east side of Peck Hill Road were influenced by Spanish architecture, as seen from the Tuscan Doric columns, French Doors and hipped clay, terracotta roofing. Buildings on the west were influenced by Tudor Style, as seen in the stucco and redwood architecture.[12]

The soaring red-brick edifices scattered amongst the vast campus composed of large ornate columns with verandas, which made it the largest of seven public tuberculosis sanitaria in the state.[13] This neo-classical, Southern plantation-style complex, designed by John Hopper Coxhead, an American architect who established the original footprint for the administration building, and the dining hall rotunda, features a circular dome with aqua walls towering up 2 ½ stories to half-moon windows and intricately stained glass that dimpled out of the ceiling. The center of the ocular dome features the Star of David with black patterned borders etched along golden-amber stained glass. Aside from patients eating here, other festivities included movies, card parties and social gatherings to help patients cope with boredom.[14] Coxhead also designed the first two patient wings, as well as, an array of other buildings along with Howard Beck.[15]

The original brick veneer buildings feature linking curved corridors that contain the common rooms and offices. At the center of the complex, the aerial orientation of Buildings #6, #2, #1, #3 and #7 look like bicycle handlebars.[16] At one point in time, a circular driveway sat beneath the entrance to the main building (Building #1).[17] Now its fissures of asphalt protrude with overgrowth and weeds when not covered in an ivory blanket of winter. A large stone stairwell still leads to the main doors with an open piazza and large Ionic columns, but the lampposts that once bore the symbol of freedom no longer flaunt their bronze eagles.

On the second and third stories to the patient wards constructed by Howard Beck (Buildings #6 and #7), open concrete loggias replaced the wooden verandas and balustrades seen in the first two wings (Buildings #2 and #3), along with reinforced metal fencing just inside the evenly spaced columns.[18] Building #44 contains the clinic, operating suite and the auditorium, some of which I explored, but other parts became unsafe and off limits due to the tremendous risk associated with snow loads and ice.[19] Building #20, built in 1923, is the powerhouse, completely separate, and off to the east of the main buildings.[20] The powerhouse introduced new boilers that replaced coal with gas, while a steam system provided heat to the buildings. This utilitarian building supplied power to the sanitarium up until 1960. Building #18 is the carpenter's shop. Other garages, tool sheds and buildings on-site still exist, but were not explored due to weather and safety, as well as buildings across Peck Hill Road, where staff housing and the director's house reside.[21] These buildings differ in style, incorporating a Tudor design with stucco and redwood throughout the architecture.

There were two construction periods, first in 1912 upon the completion of the complex, and again in 1924 to 1928 to add additions. Rehabilitation of buildings also took place from 1933 to 1936 and housing upgrades took place in 1952, adding Buildings #46 to #53.[22] Renovations and maintenance did not happen again until 1965 and over the span of thirty-four years to 1989, more than forty projects took place, requiring the upwards of $7.5 million.[23]

Popular local legend says Mayor James Noble Adam donated this dome from the Hall of Music acquired at the 1901 Pan-American Exposition in Buffalo, NY. It was under this dome that President McKinley was assassinated, but there is no verifiable proof to support either of these allegations.

Up until 1960, the J. N. Adam Memorial Hospital was utilized as a tuberculosis sanitarium and for its first thirty-six years of operations, it was run by the City of

Buffalo. In 1948, a deed transferred the property back to New York State, with a Reverter Clause to the City of Buffalo.[24] The hospital held two directors in its time as a tuberculosis sanitarium: Dr. Clarence Hyde from 1912-1921 and Dr. Horace LoGrasso from 1921-1948.[25]

The hospital briefly shut down in 1960 and reopened that September as a mental health facility for developmental disabilities and functioned as a subsidiary of Gowanda State Hospital. By 1972, the facility changed its name to J. N. Adam Developmental Center and became an independent facility, again operating under the New York State Department of Mental Hygiene.

> In 1985, J. N. Adam Developmental Center received an award for being the most energy efficient of twenty-two office centers for Mental Retardation and Developmental Disabilities that operated in New York State at that time.[26]

By 1991, it ceased operations as an institutional treatment facility, withering away as a derelict piece of forgotten history.[27] This complex holds a plethora of untold stories and memories as Buffalo's first municipal tuberculosis hospital, where several patients were healed and lived on to shape the economy, molding Western New York into what it now is today.

The non-profit "Friends of J. N. Adam" tried to preserve the hospital, inviting the public to join in their efforts of saving this historical masterpiece. They searched for a reuse of the buildings, along with protecting its 649 acres of forests, meadows, streams, ponds and milieu, sitting on the town's abundant water supply.[28] With the original aquifer providing a capacity of one half million gallons of water to the hospital, and, in 1924, an additional one million gallon reservoir added, totaling a capacity of 1.5 million gallons, you can understand why this non-profit fought so hard for its preservation and restoration.[29] Even with the 469 signatures acquired from an online petition (now Change.org), their dream of preserving and protecting the land along with the restoration of these architectural treasures never happened.[30] Although many allegations speculated its listing on the NYS Register of Historic Places in 1985, this was also a myth. According to Jennifer Walkowski, the property was reviewed in the 1980s for eligibility of historic listing, but the appropriate documentation was never forwarded to New York State or the National Registrar of Historic Places.[31]

In 2005, city and state officials wanted to sell the hospital to Trathen Land Co. logging company for $371,000, but as NY solicited bids for the second time in the building's history, discrepancies between state and the City of Buffalo halted the sale.[32]

Efforts to repurpose the damaged land from the abandonment of the J. N. Adam Memorial Hospital took place up until the year 2013 by a local non-profit organization, which tried to preserve the native trees, birds, and other species in the environment, but their efforts remained futile because of the tremendous costs associated with any reuse or repurposing. This still left the community of Perrysburg scrambling to find a solution of what to do with the derelict buildings occupying 649 acres. Aside from being an eyesore and a public health risk because of the lead, asbestos, mold and other toxic substances on-site, it has become inherently dangerous and more unsafe over the years and continues to attract attention from vandals and trespassers.

In 2015, Senator Catharine Young proposed a bill allocating a budget of $235,000 to fund a study for redevelopment potential of the former J. N. Adam Memorial Hospital. Originally, Governor Cuomo vetoed the bill on November 20, 2015, due to lack of funding. The bill would have provided consulting costs to cover the study of the hospital. Almost a year later the bill passed.[33]

In 2017, the appraisal of the New York State Office of General Services' marketing and redevelopment study for the J. N. Adam Memorial Hospital assessed the land at $880,000. However, with demolition and inherent on-site environmental issues due in part to gross negligence, from its unmaintained, rotting state, it was estimated to cost $3.8 to $14.6 million. Reuse of the current buildings estimated in the ballpark of $15.6 to $18 million.[34] So neither option appeared viable—even if the state gave it away for free, not one developer would consider touching this project due to its calamity! Her buildings will continue to melt away through the seasons until the roofs disappear to clouds of brick, and her walls wither away to piles of laden rubble.

To this day J. N. Adam Memorial Hospital crumbles in one of the most immaculate pastoral settings of Perrysburg, NY, overlooking deep green coniferous forests and farmland with a glimpse of deep blue Lake Erie beyond the rolling hillside of the Allegheny Mountains. It's no wonder the county's slogan "Enchanted Mountains" fit this historical gem so beautifully.[35] The site still struggles today with its battle of ownership between the City of Buffalo and New York State while it continues to suffer Mother Nature's tumultuous hymns of brutal winters and monstrous storms.

As I wander the relics of dusty decay, I wonder what stories and memories are held within her dilapidated walls. How many patients were saved from tuberculosis? Who lived to see her demise? What will happen to this forgotten piece of history that is slowly crumbling away in the small town of Perrysburg? I can only dream and fill in the gaps of her past with soft memories of her potential future.

BUILDING #1 – THE MAIN BUILDING

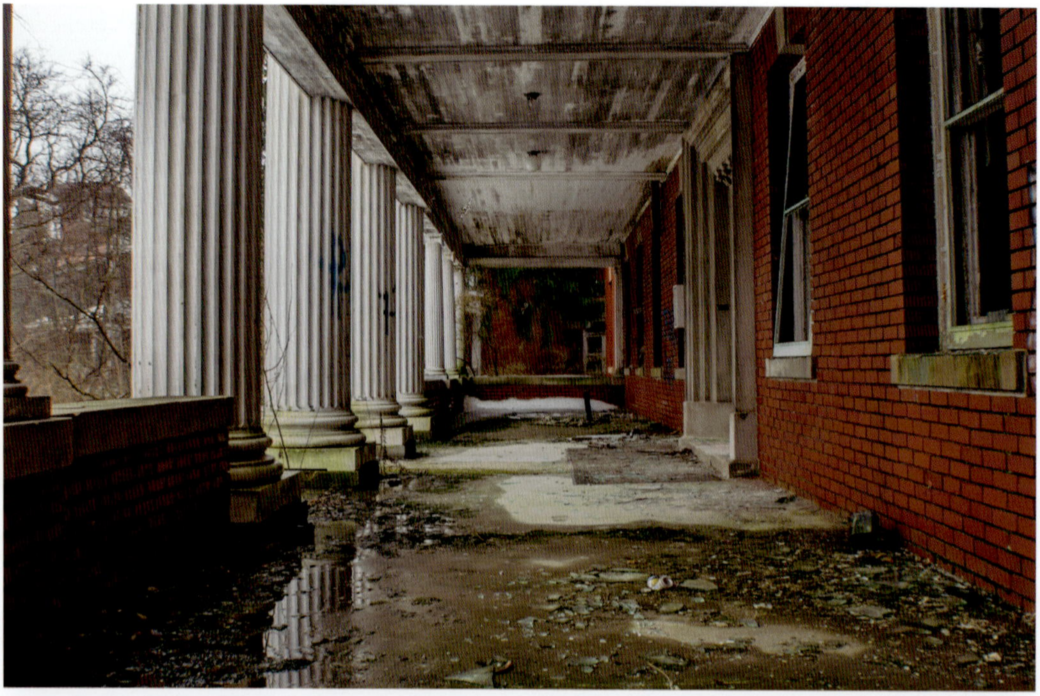

As I gaze down the row of Tuscan Doric columns, I catch a glimpse of what's to come. *[Photo by Brian Cray]*

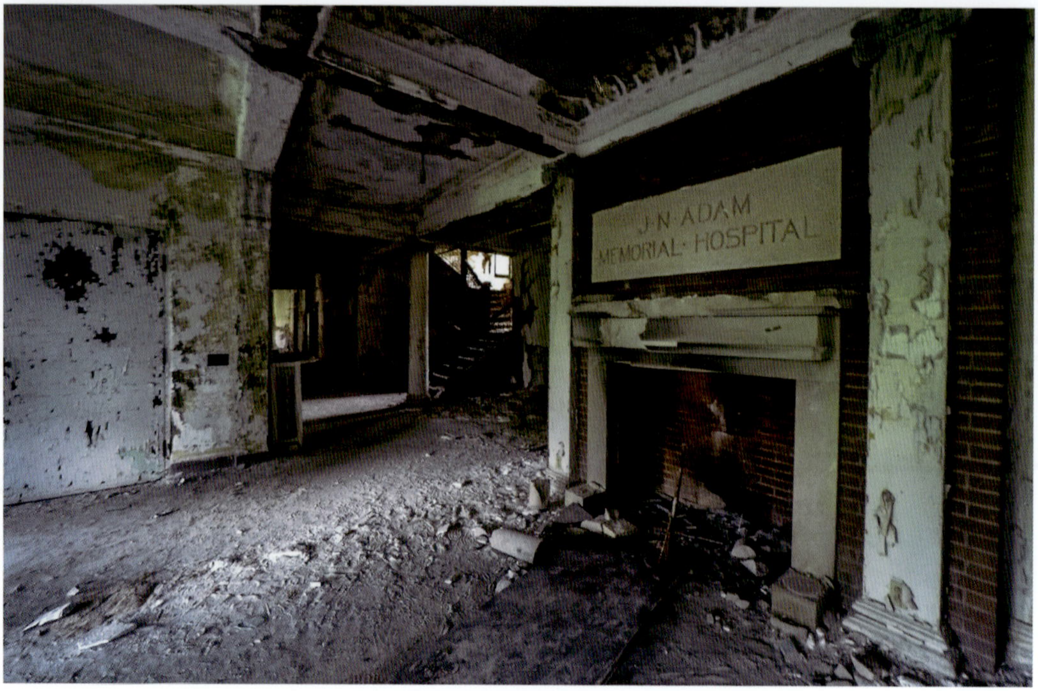

In 2016, from the very first time I cast my eyes on the crumbling façade I wanted to know her story. *[Photo by Brian Cray]*

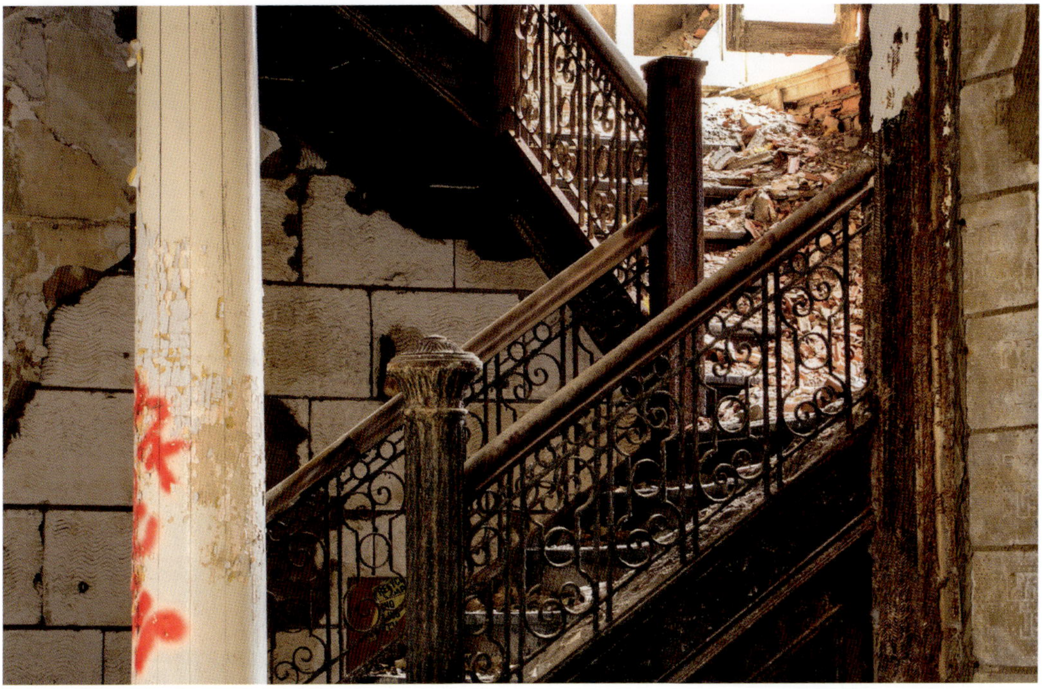

I gaze at banisters soaring to the heavens, zigzagging up decrepit walls, and beyond the freckles of decay rest heaps of splintered bricks. They slowly tumble with age, and the graceful gusts of Mother Nature, hoping to rid themselves of her dying walls. *[Photo by Brian Cray]*

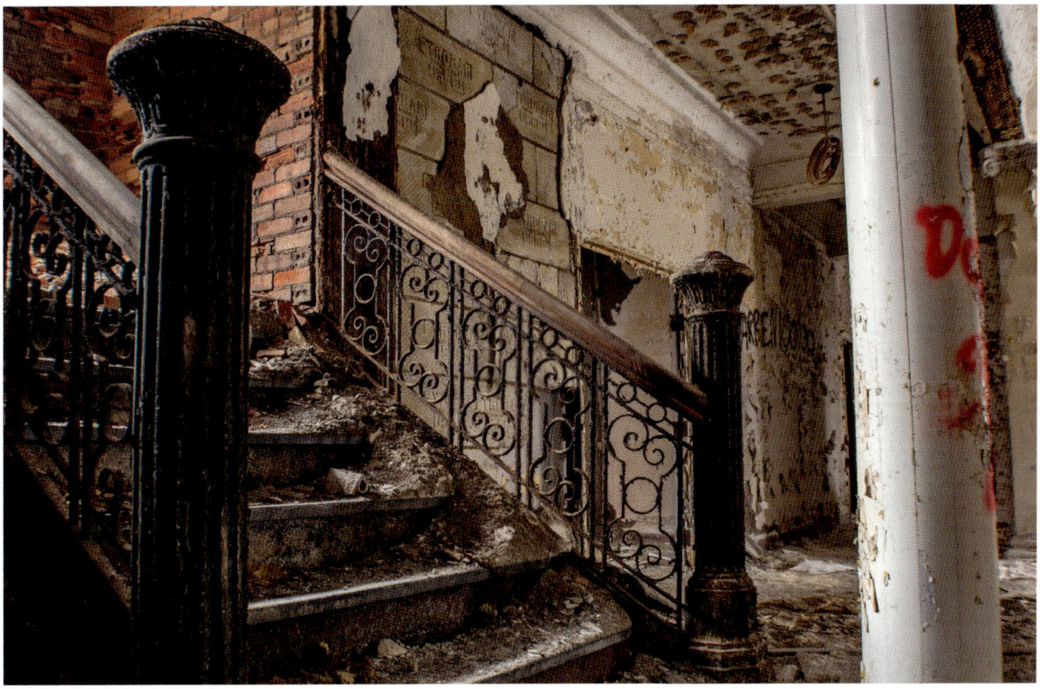

The rungs pile pillows of dust in each corner as scabs of wounds flake off from her walls. Still she is beautiful despite the plague of decay. *[Photo by Brian Cray]*

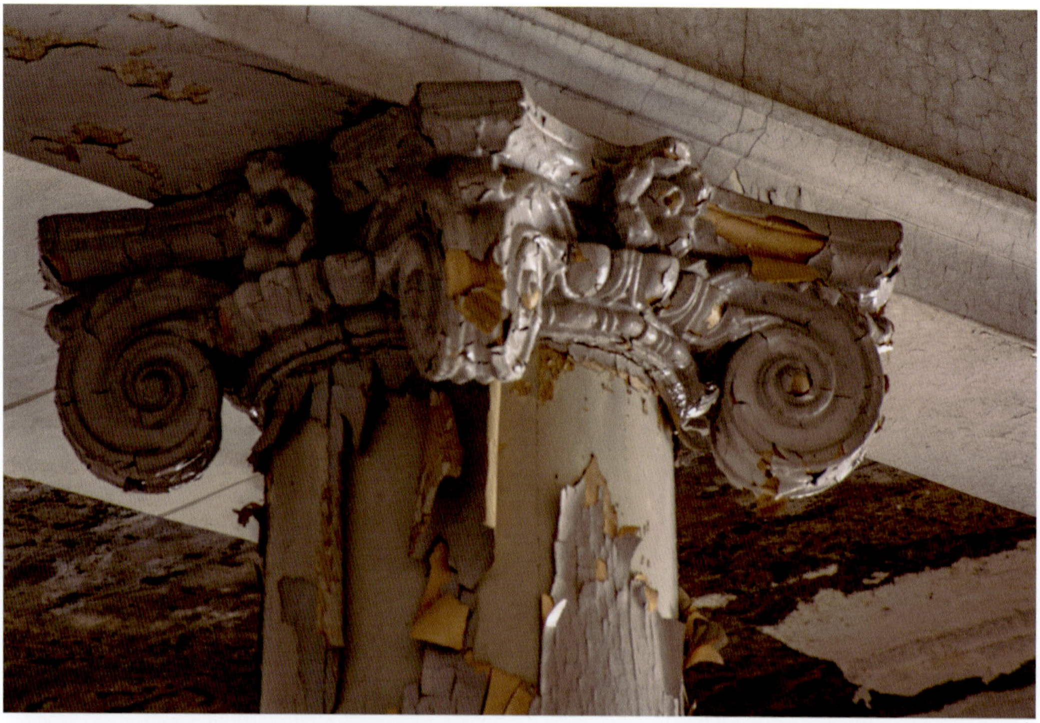

Exquisite columns still tower, ceilings robust in stature beneath their peeling skin. *[Photo by Brian Cray]*

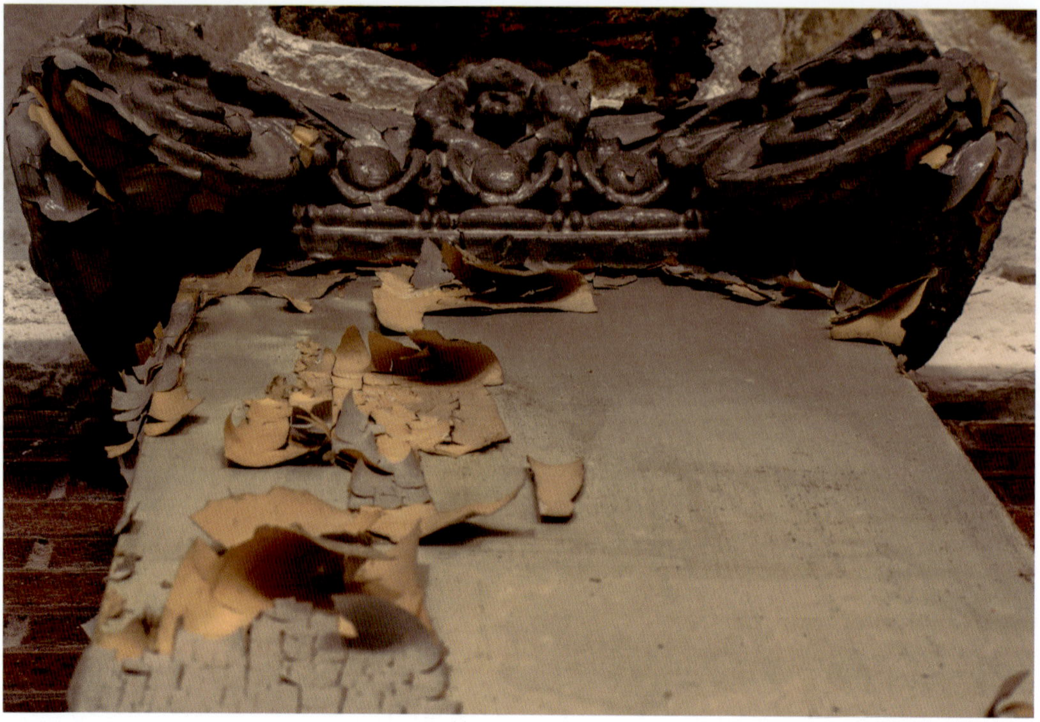

Asbestos flakes off every column and wall, contaminating the land on which she decays, hindering the site valueless. *[Photo by Brian Cray]*

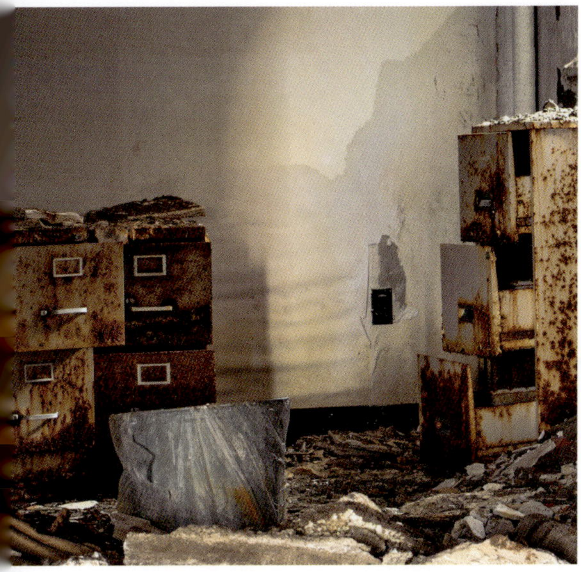

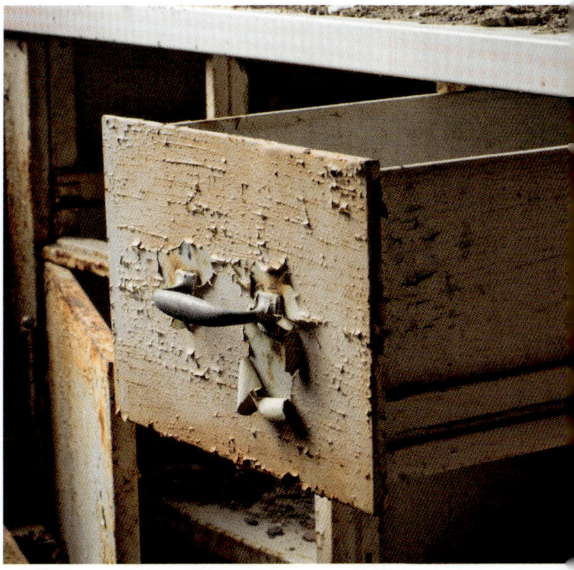

Above left: It's as if one day everyone left, and never came back, leaving medical documents and furnishings behind to rot over the decades. *[Photo by Brian Cray]*

Above right: What did these empty drawers once hold? Patient medical files, research on the application of light—we can only speculate. But, within these walls Dr. Brian O'Brien scribbled notes, inventing arc lamps for the sun cure during winter months, while administering the irradiation of milk for vitamin D (Siegmund). *[Photo by Brian Cray]*

Below: As I creep slowly through her shell, I see another lone chair. This thinking chair will change from room to room. I close my eyes and try to swoop in on the past. What did she look like before time strangled her beauty? *[Photo by Brian Cray]*

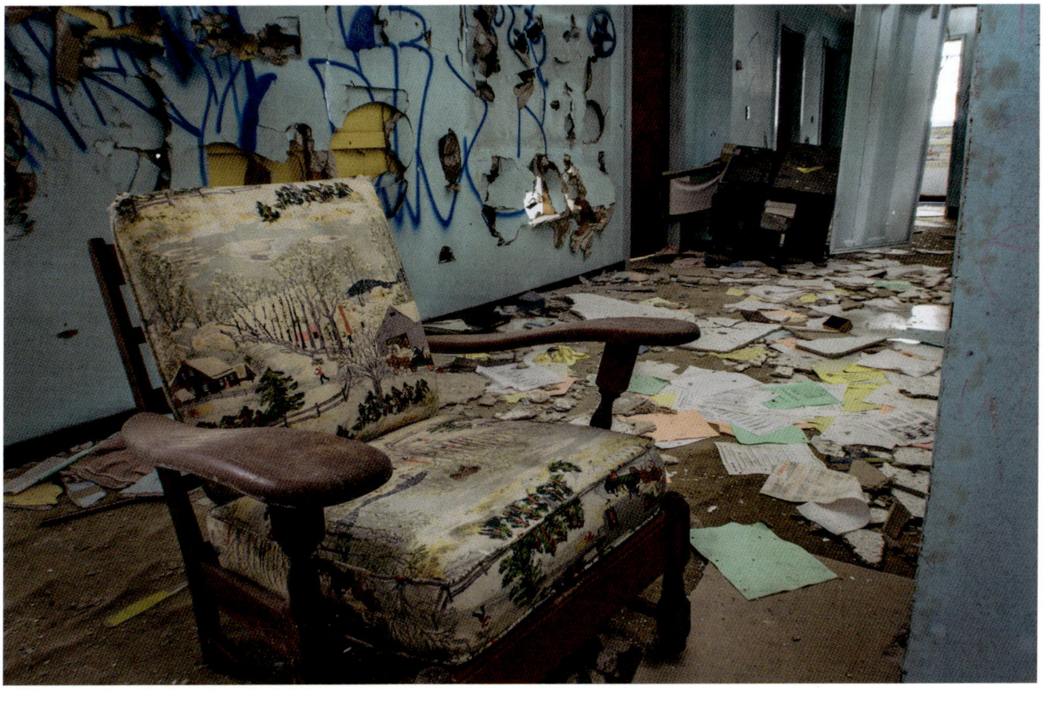

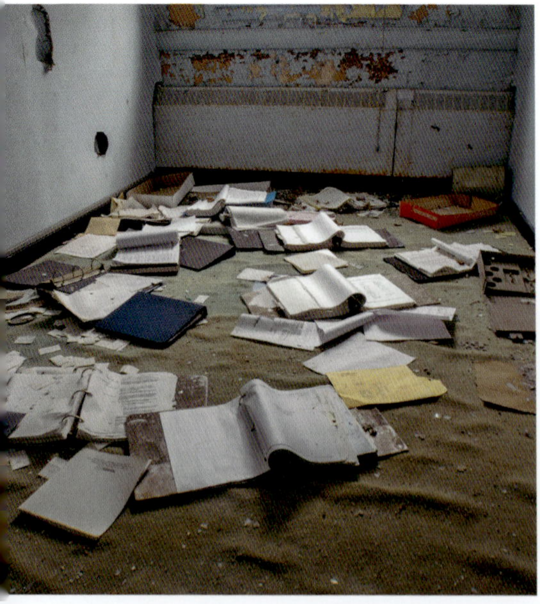

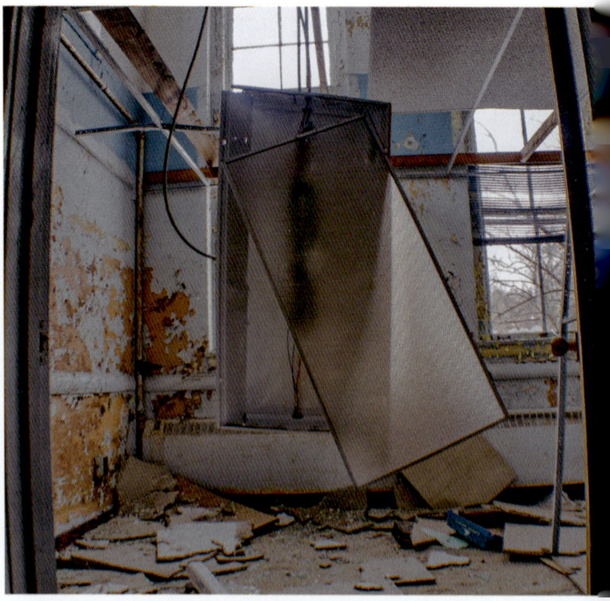

Above left: Scattered binders, notebooks and loose papers tell the stories of the patients who once walked inside these walls. *[Photo by Brian Cray]*

Above right: A busted light fixture dangles by a small thread of wire as it hangs from the ceiling like a noose. I stop and lock my eyes on it before wandering the halls to the kitchen. *[Photo by Brian Cray]*

Below: Even the paint to the tarnished kilns fades away at the hands of Mother Nature. *[Photo by Brian Cray]*

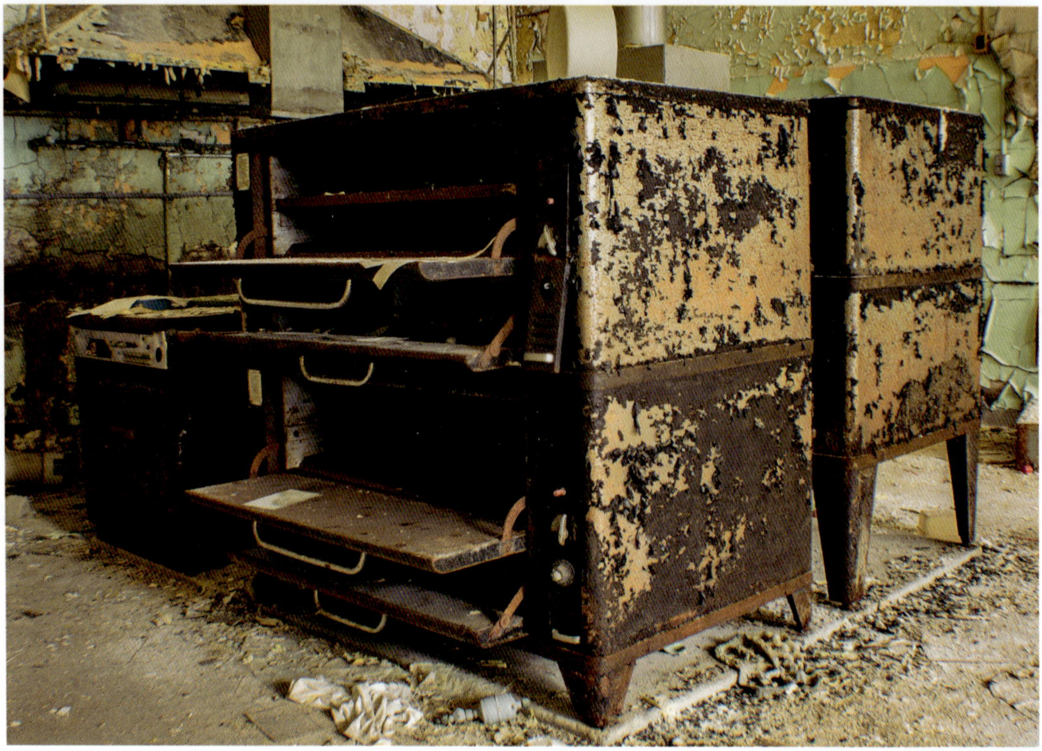

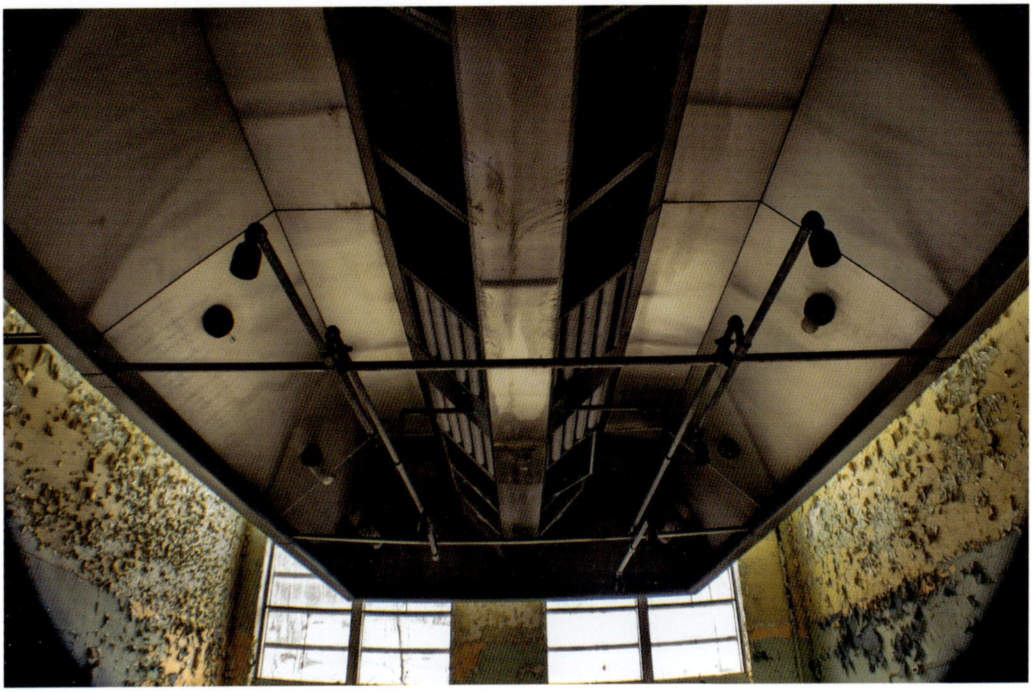

As I look through the wide-angle lens of my camera I see the sheen silver glint from the stainless steel hood. It looks pristine, but it's not until my eyes drift to the walls that I see otherwise. *[Photo by Brian Cray]*

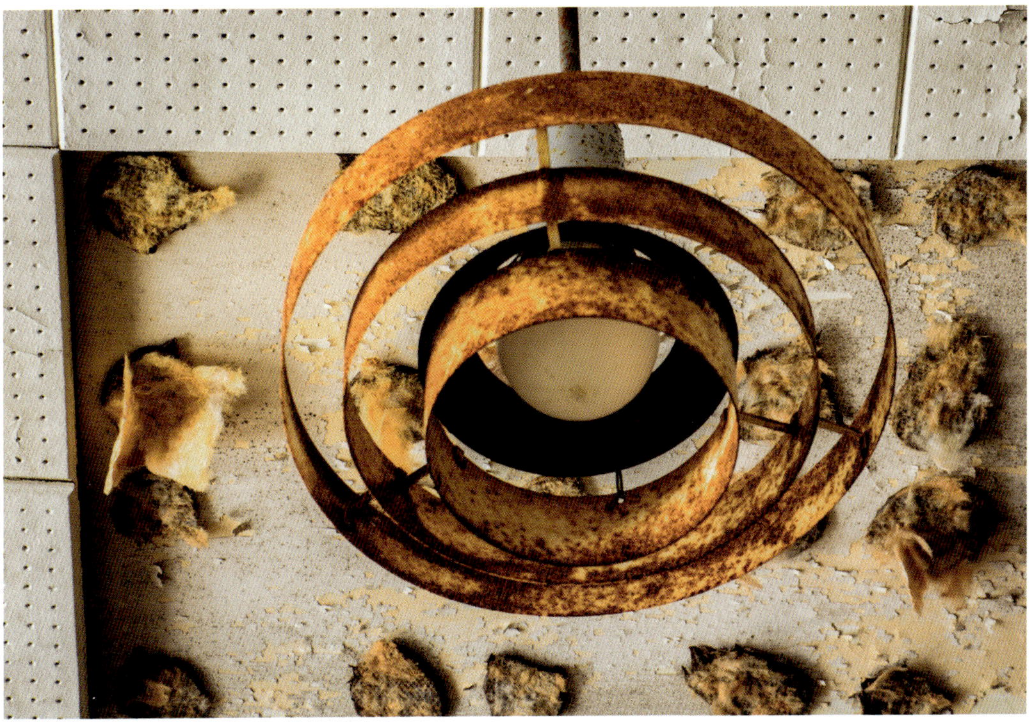

A lamp hangs plastered with rust. Behind it glue grips pieces of insulation left behind from fallen ceiling tiles as I drift closer to the stained-glass dome of the dining hall rotunda. *[Photo by Brian Cray]*

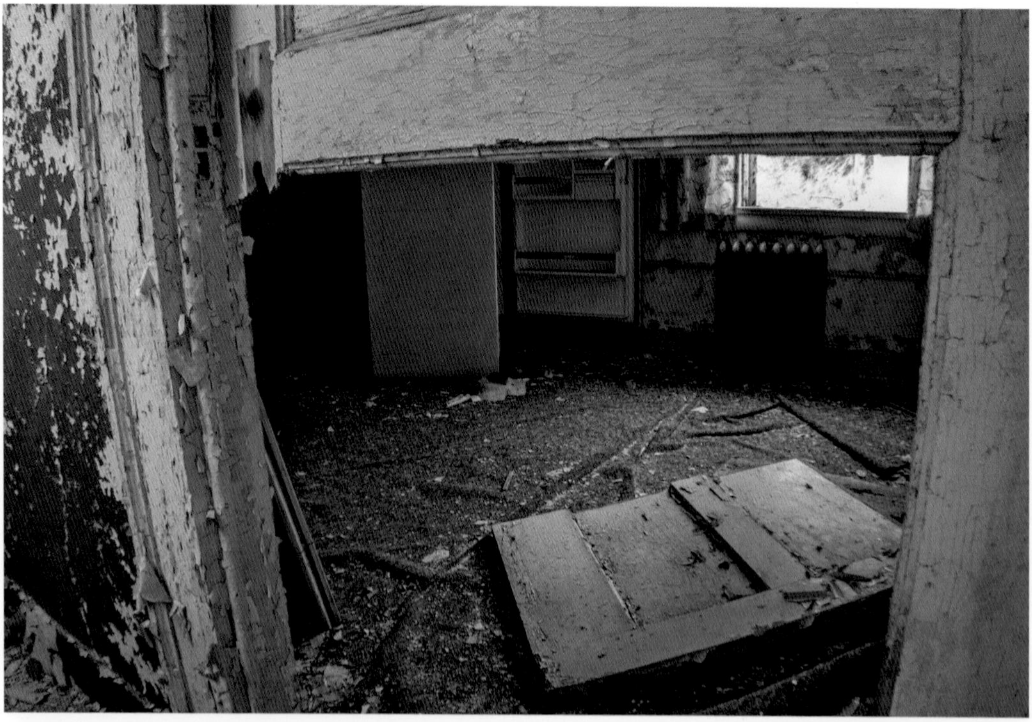

As I peep through a half-broken door frame, my eyes lock onto the splintered bits of wood that blend with the ruffles of shag carpet in a patient wing. *[Photo by Brian Cray]*

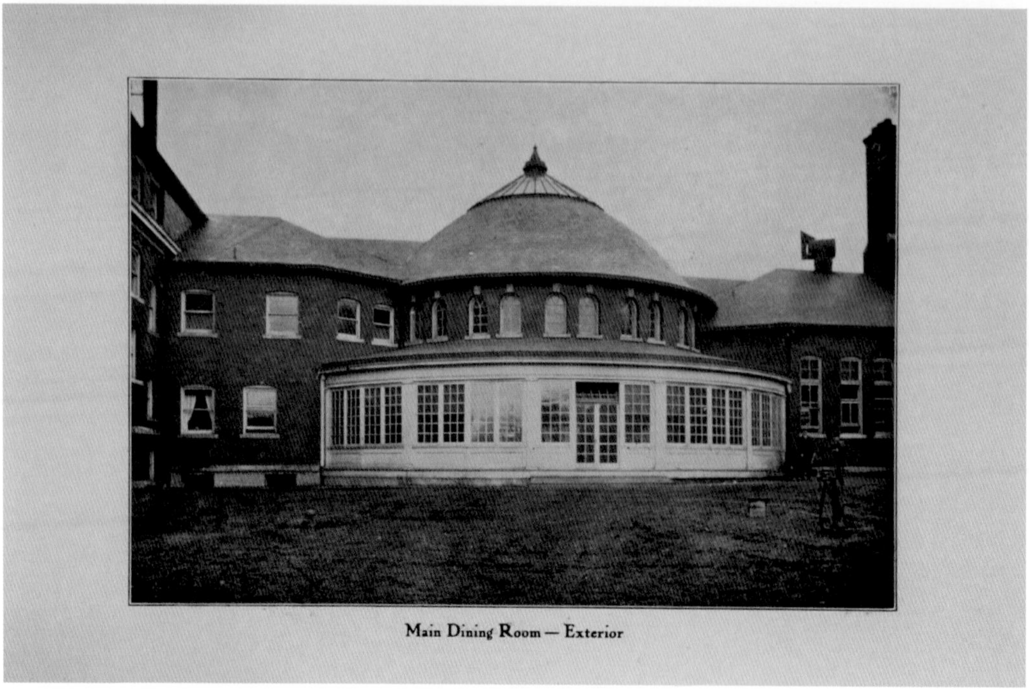

Curved glass invites the sunshine into the dining hall rotunda, but through the years the wall has changed to blood-red bricks, slowly hemorrhaging with time. *[Photo by Frank Ruslander, 1920]*

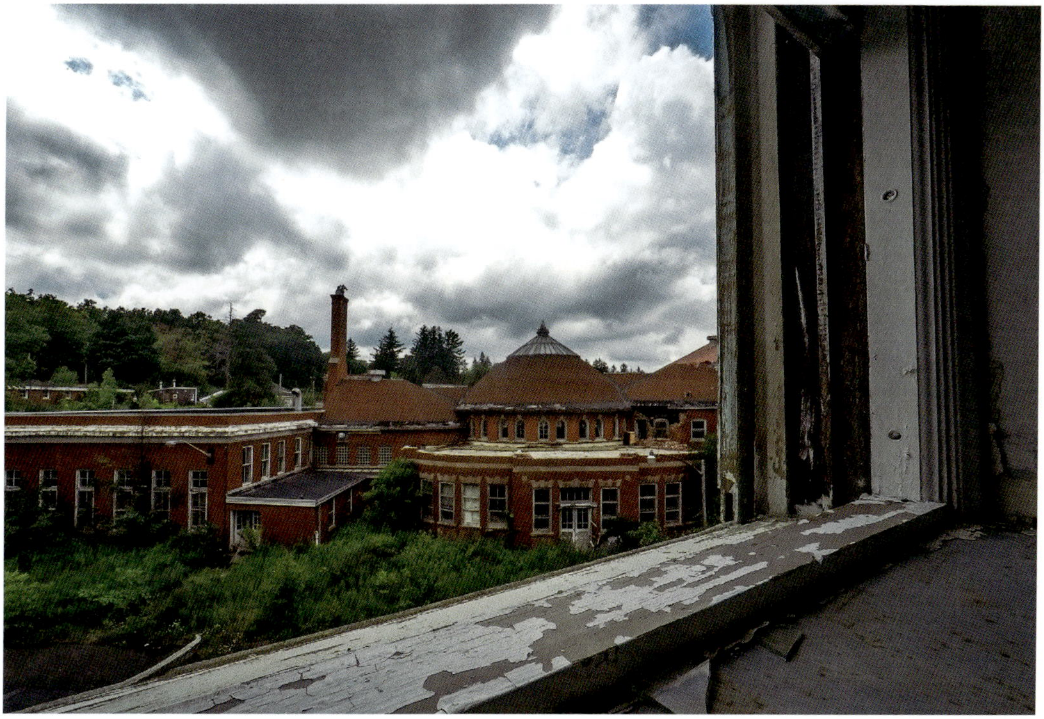

Flash forward almost 100 years later and you can see the rehabilitations that were done to the curved façade. *[Photo by Brian Cray]*

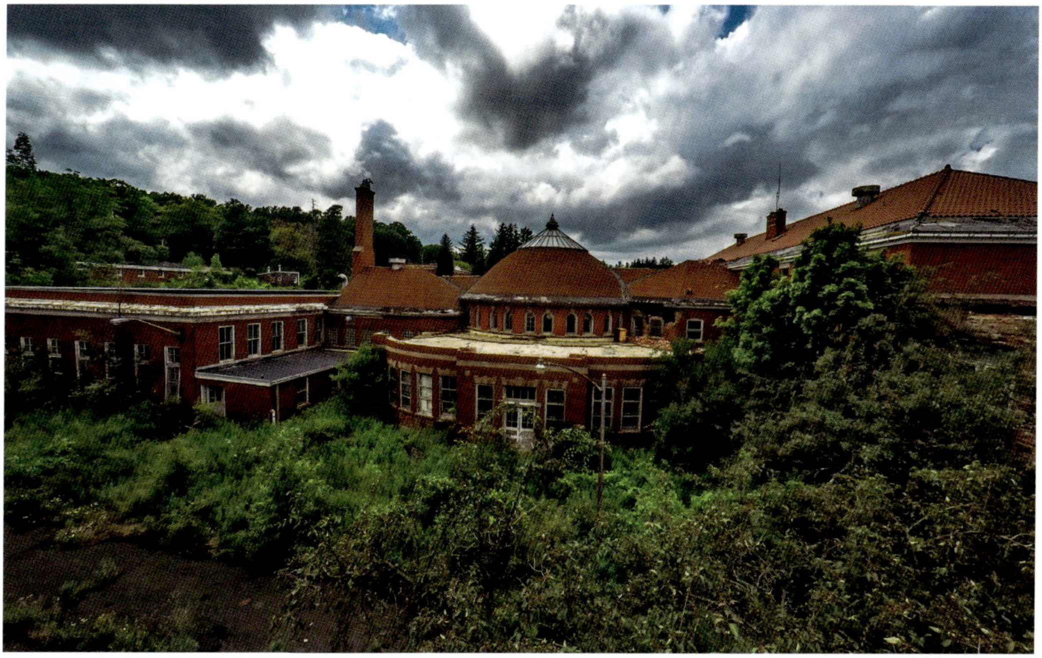

From the backside of the administration building I stand among a rusted stairwell. I glance out at the ocular dome to the dining hall rotunda where patients once ate, played cards and gathered for social events. This was my first time exploring the hospital in 2016. *[Photo by Brian Cray]*

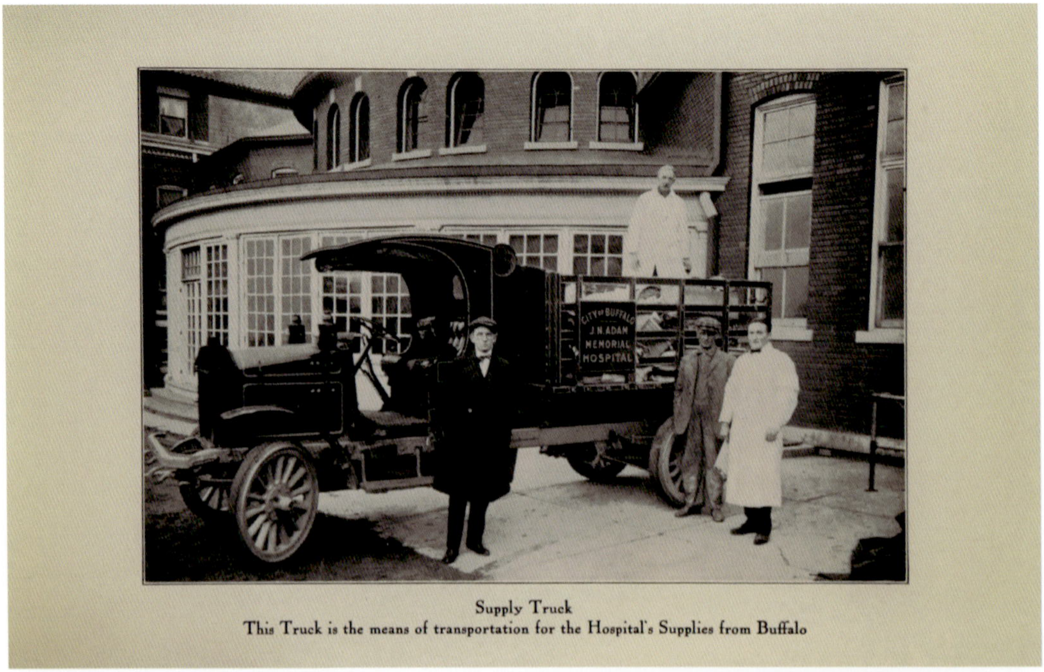

Supply Truck
This Truck is the means of transportation for the Hospital's Supplies from Buffalo

[Photo by Frank Ruslander, 1920]

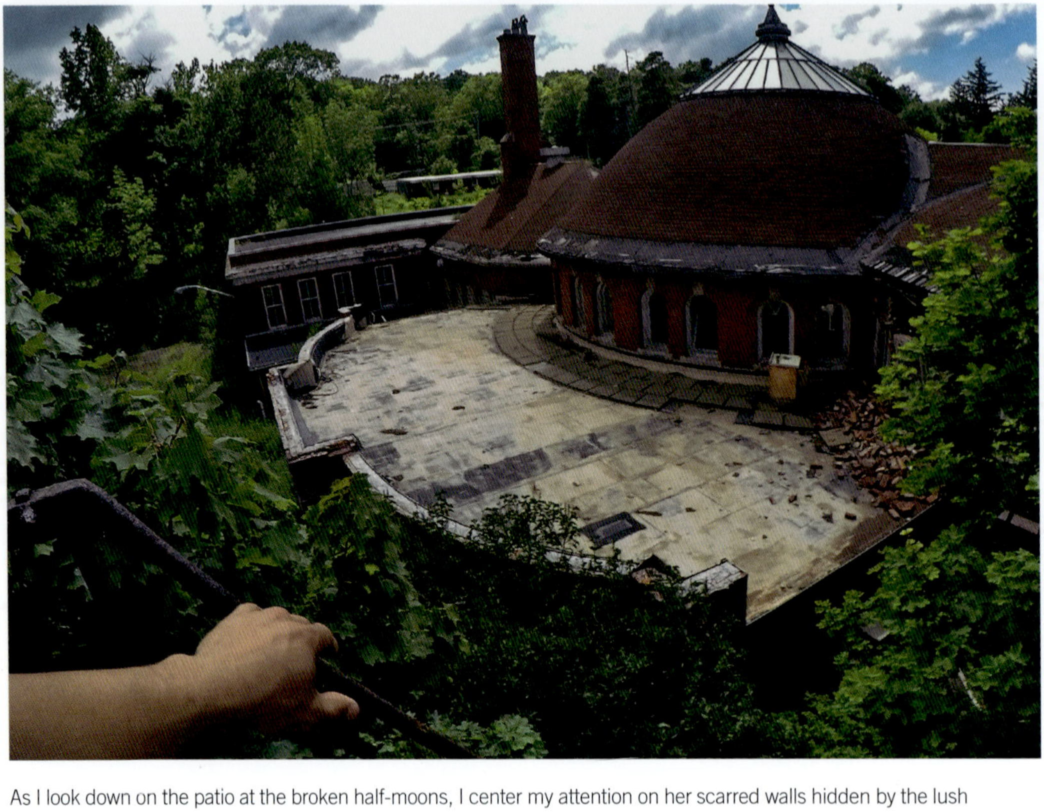

As I look down on the patio at the broken half-moons, I center my attention on her scarred walls hidden by the lush forest in the corner. What will come of the stained glass behind the curving walls of her dome? *[Photo by Brian Cray]*

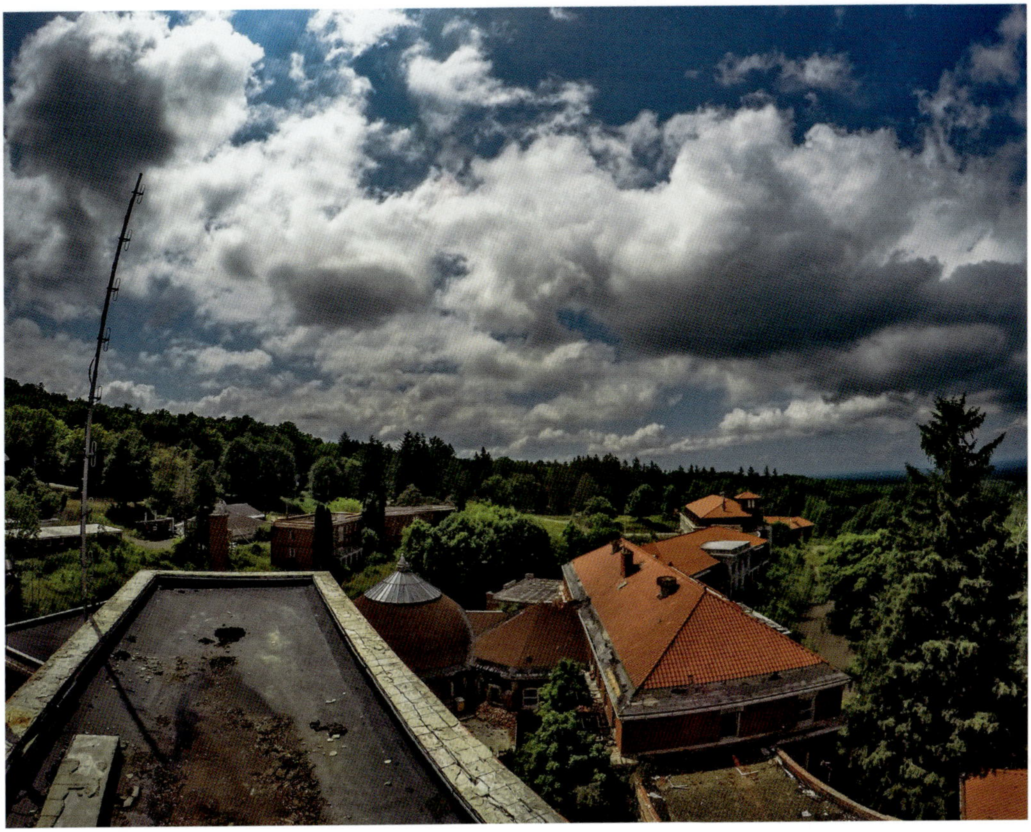

As I wander the flat roof of Building #44, I look out across the complex on this clear spring day in 2016. Her bright red, hipped clay, roof tiles radiate in the sun and for a second her fate vanishes from my thoughts. *[Photo by Brian Cray]*

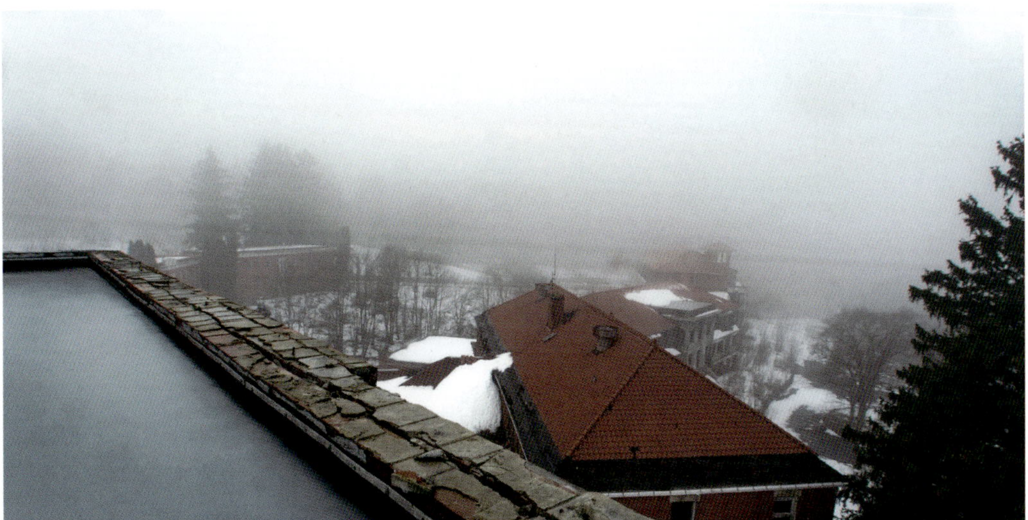

Two harsh winters since my last visit rip apart the aggregate from the curb exposing the brick along the roof of Building #44. I stand on an ice rink overlooking the main buildings in a surreal setting of fog and snow. *[Photo by Brian Cray]*

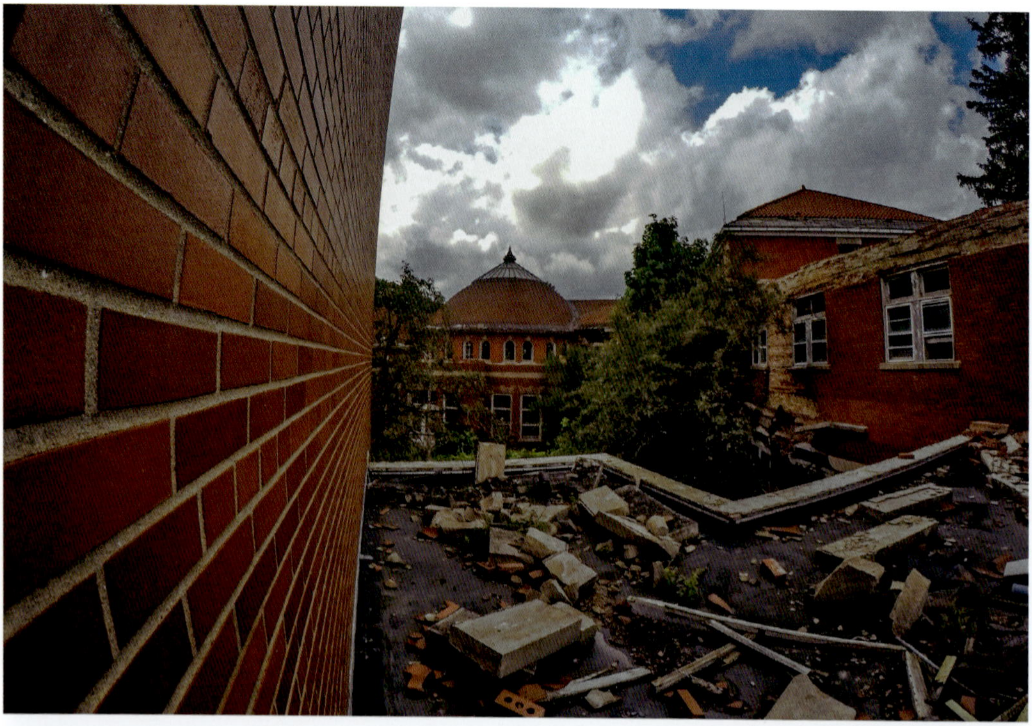

The dining hall shines in a different light these days. Follow the grout along the brick façade. Beyond the overgrowth, her curving walls hold your eyes on the nipple, under which her oculus draws in the sun through fragmented glass. *[Photo by Brian Cray]*

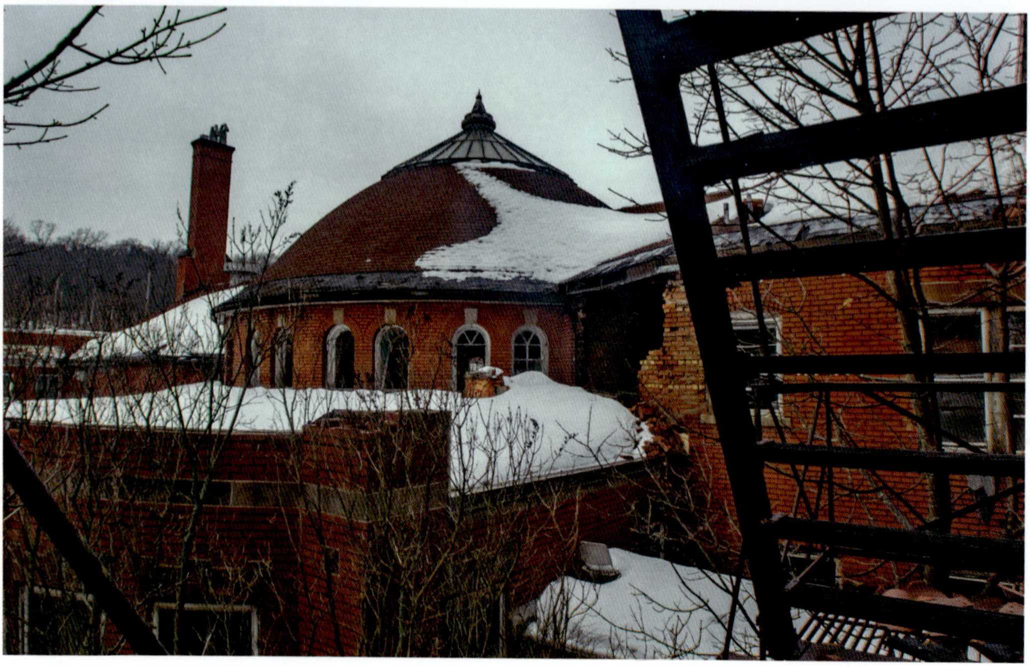

Decades of winters chisel the roof open to water damage and collapse. As I latch onto the rusted banister, I can't help but focus on her dark open wound. *[Photo by Brian Cray]*

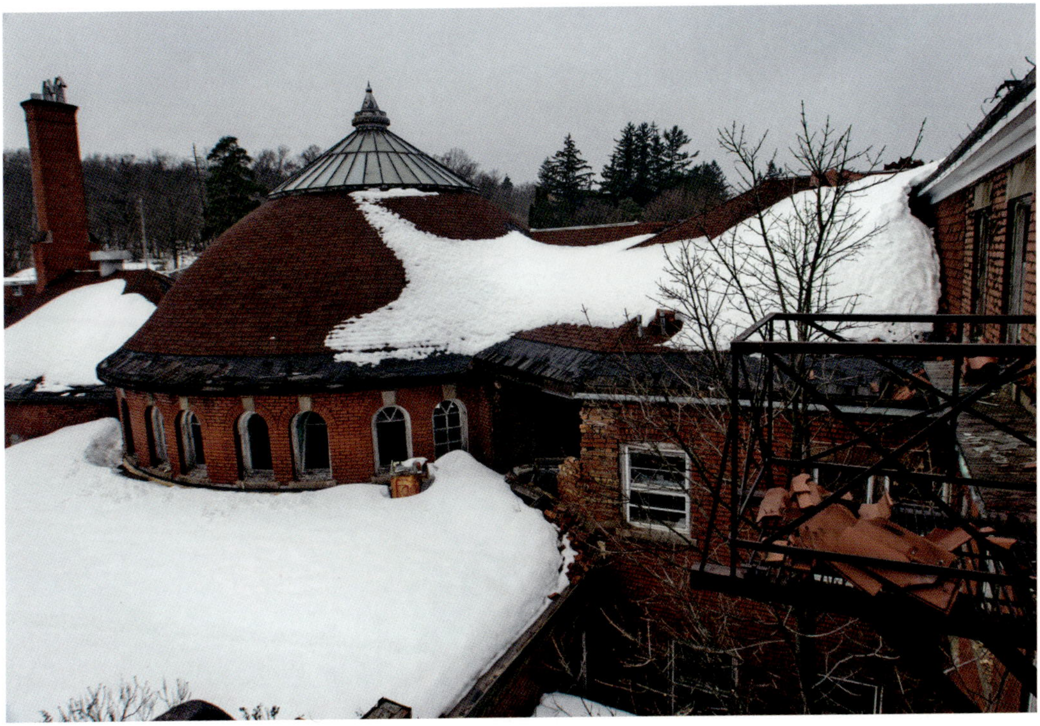

There is no repairing the walls for she has suffered far too from the severity of long winters and cold nights. *[Photo by Brian Cray]*

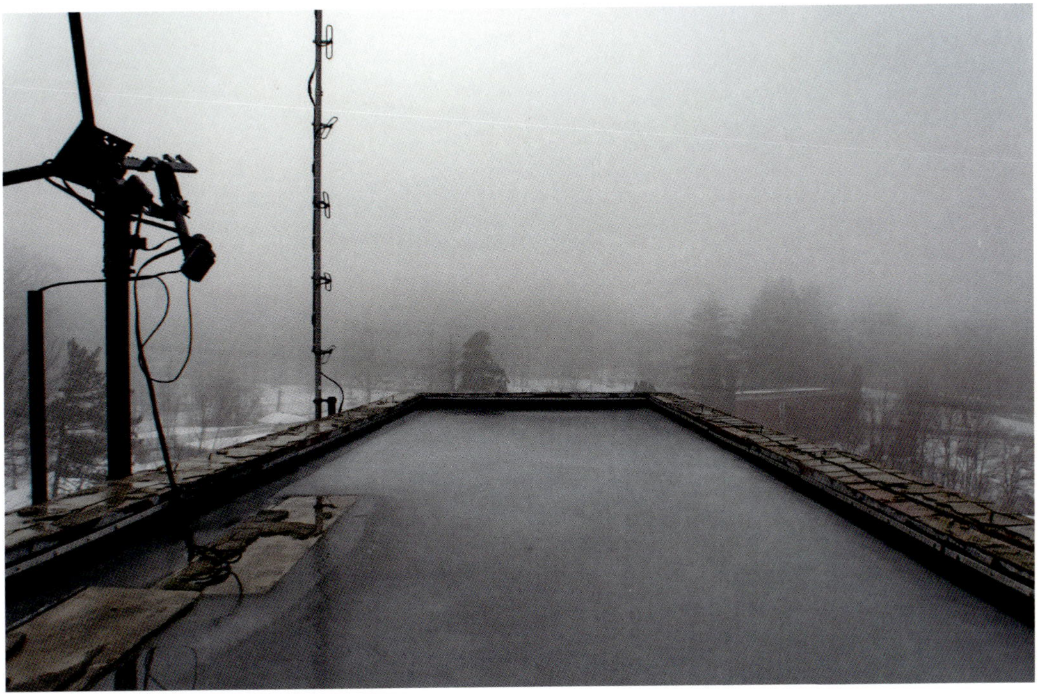

Four to six inches of ice glistens beneath me and I can only hope my added weight does not send me hurdling through the roof. *[Photo by Brian Cray]*

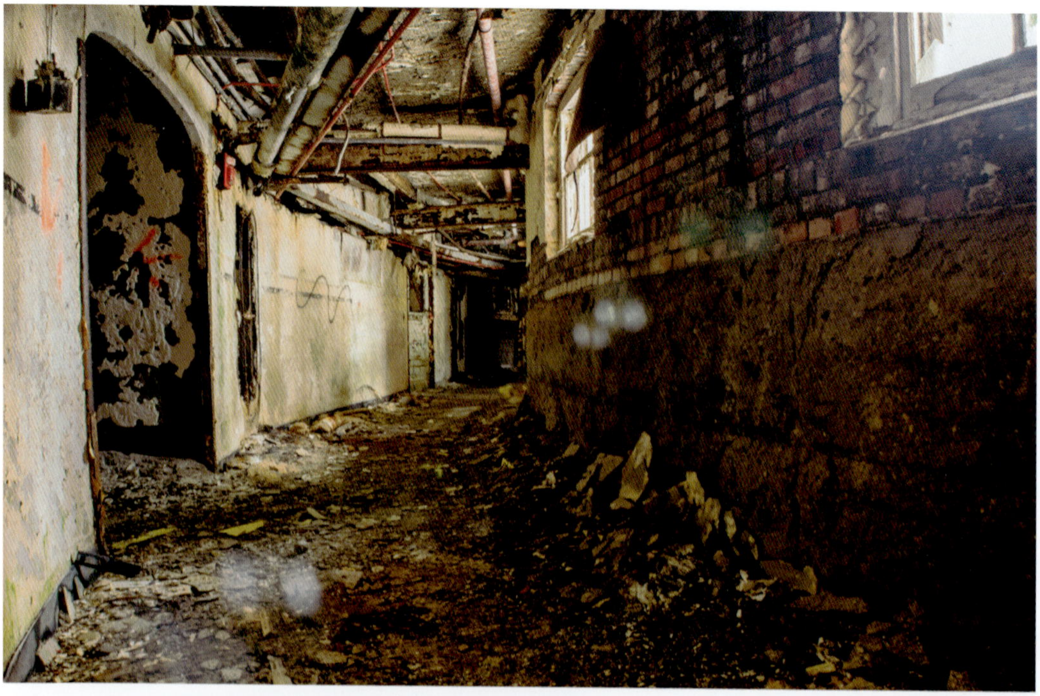

Each corridor is only a shell of the past, memories smeared along the putrefied floor. I wander deeper to get to her heart which stopped beating long ago. *[Photo by Brian Cray]*

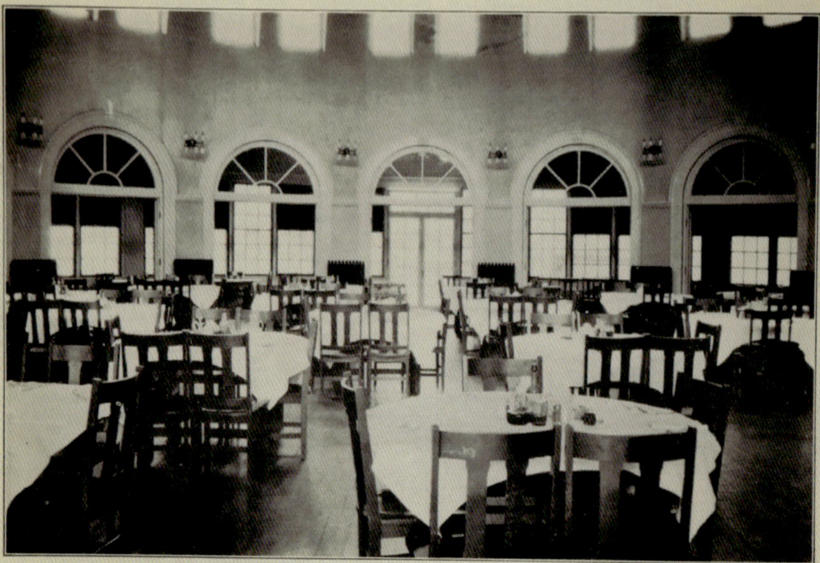

Section of Main Dining Room for Patients. One of the most beautiful Dining Rooms in the Country
Seats 200 Patients

This is the dining hall rotunda in the main building. *[Photo by Frank Ruslander, 1920]*

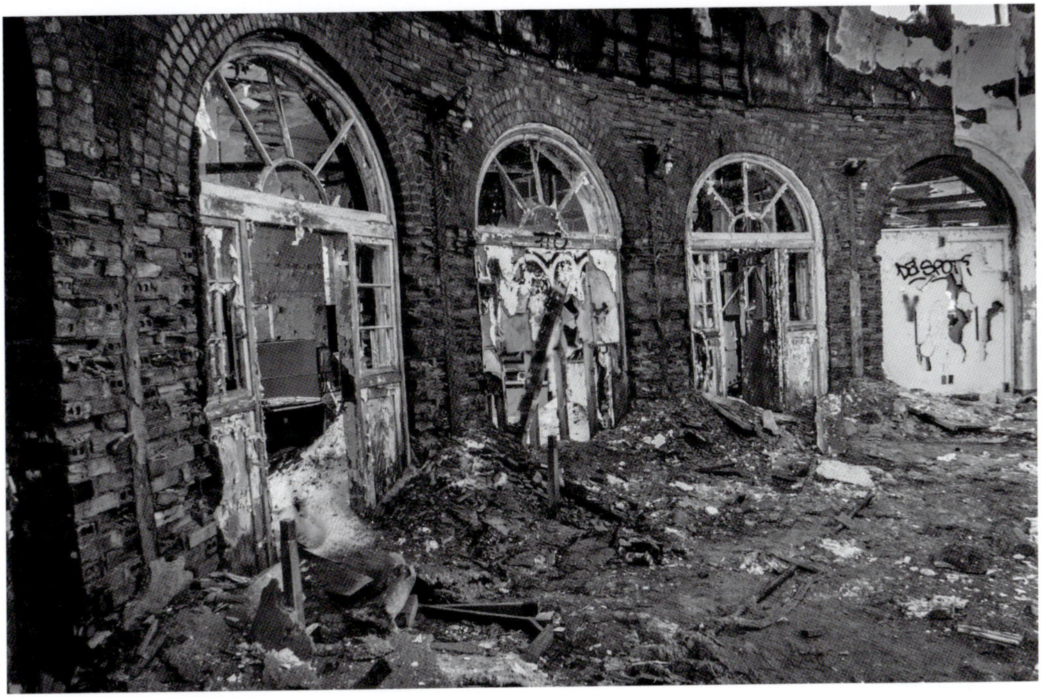

The cold fingertips of Mother Nature wrenched the plaster and paint from her walls. Now she disintegrates in heaps amongst the floor, bricks and grout join the rubble with the change of the seasons. *[Photo by Brian Cray]*

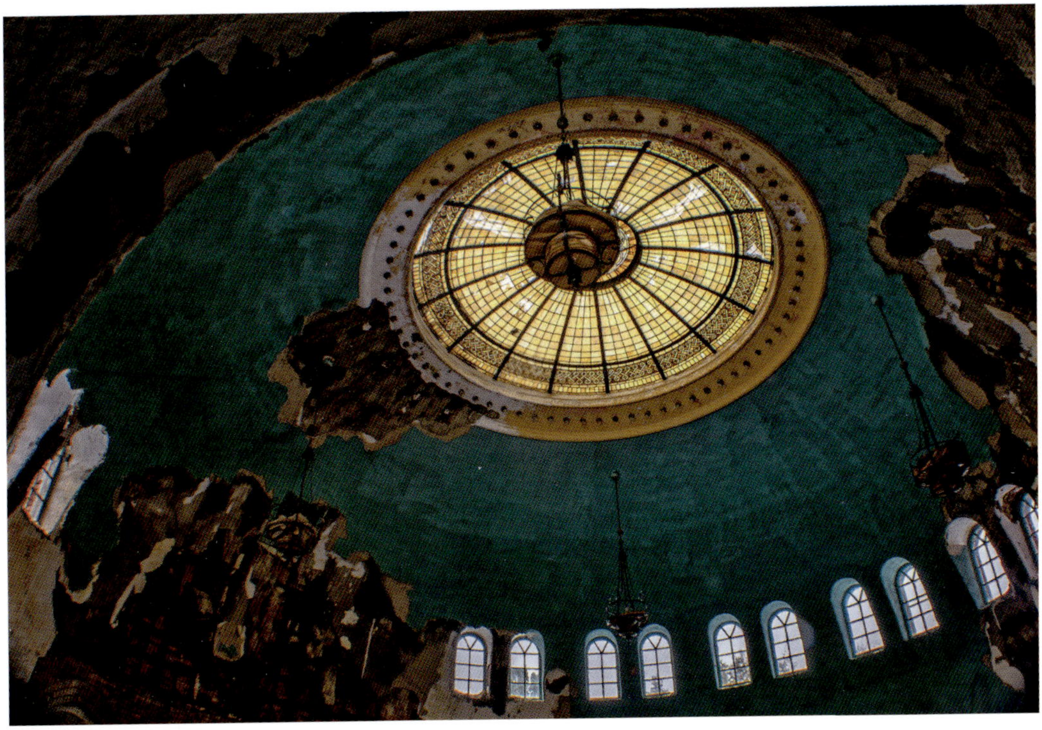

I stand between her dying arch as I look up at her chandelier masking the Star of David from the stained-glass dome. *[Photo by Brian Cray]*

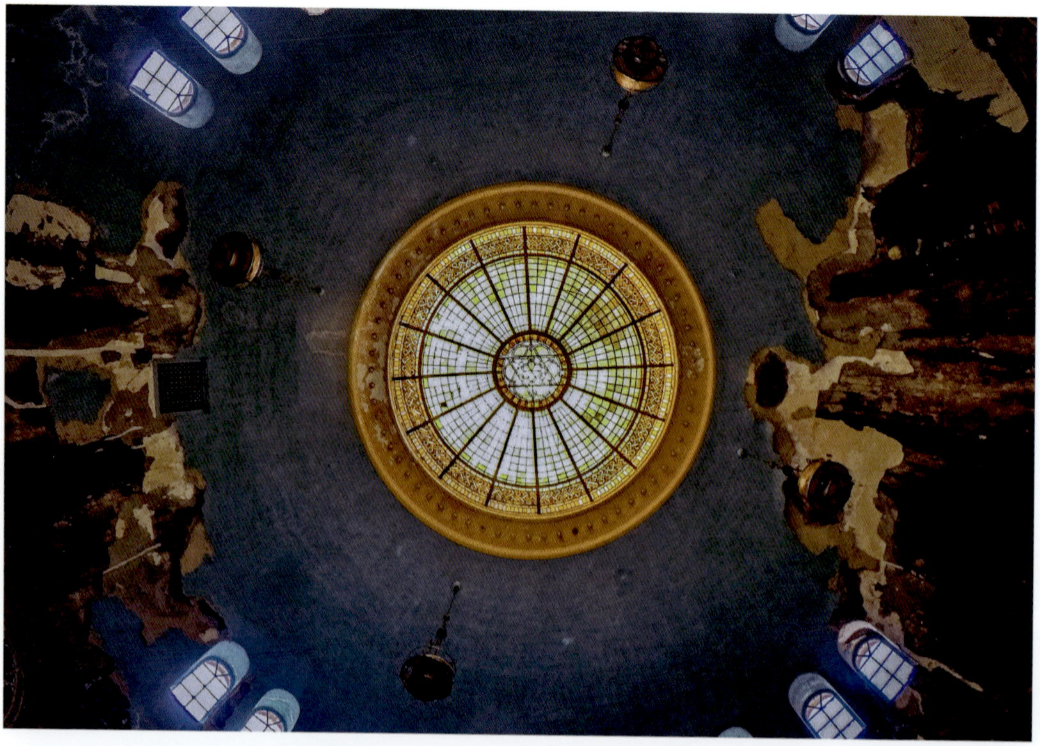

Just two years prior, on my first visit to this mystifying place, I notice how her peeling walls have not quite reached the yellow oculus. *[Photo by Brian Cray]*

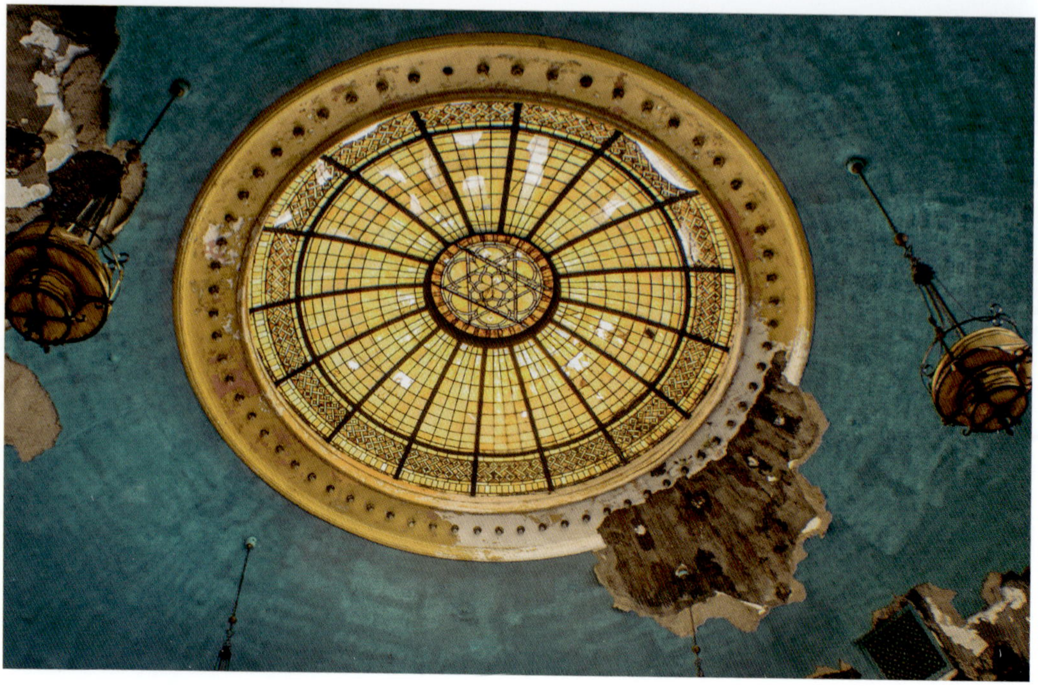

Peel back the ocean walls with the rain and snow. Soon the translucent white and golden glass will stain the floor with shattered fragments of decay. *[Photo by Brian Cray]*

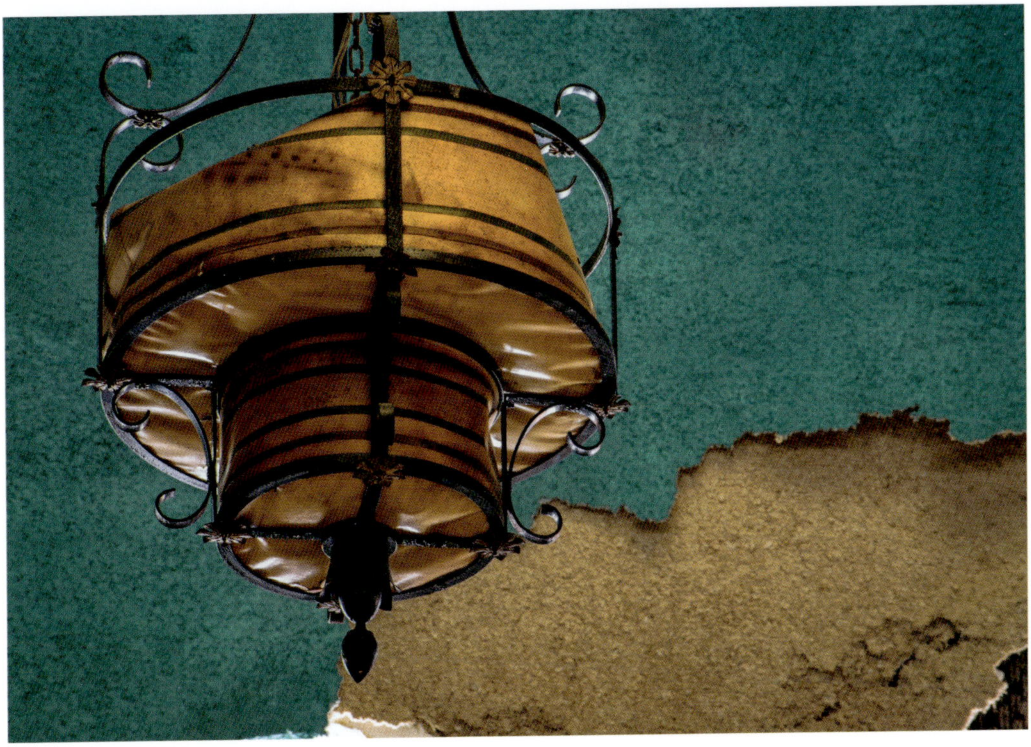

The encrusted lesions plaguing her walls slowly tear back ocean paint. They expose, scars while chandeliers sag from the ceiling awaiting their inevitable fate. *[Photo by Brian Cray]*

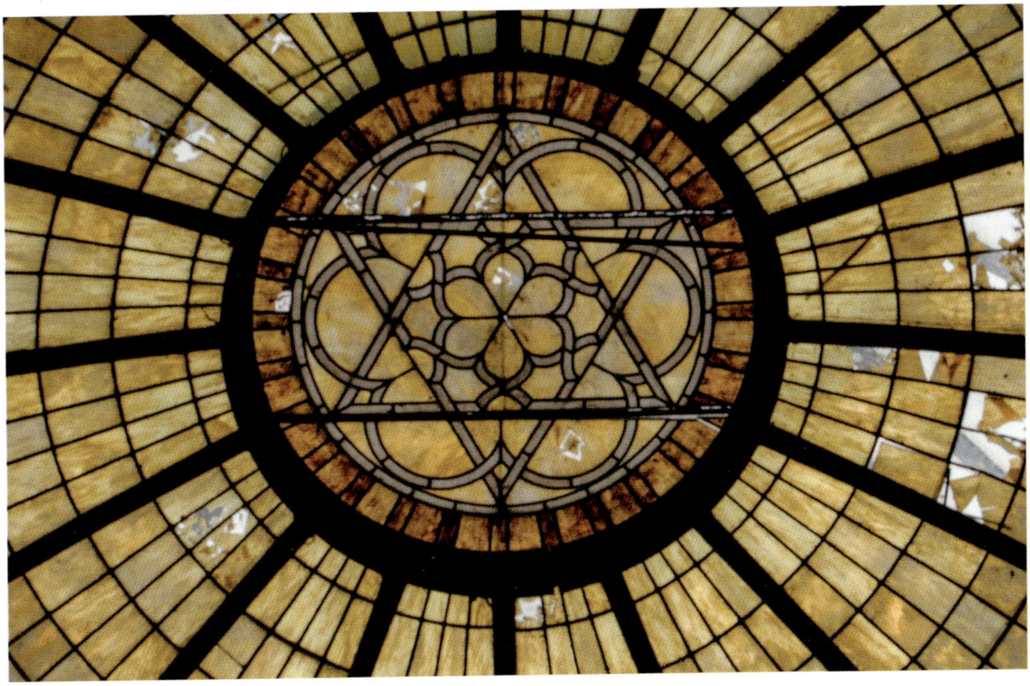

The Star of David is slowly falling victim from the ultraviolet light. The same beams of light that once raised these walls now slowly deteriorate them. *[Photo by Brian Cray]*

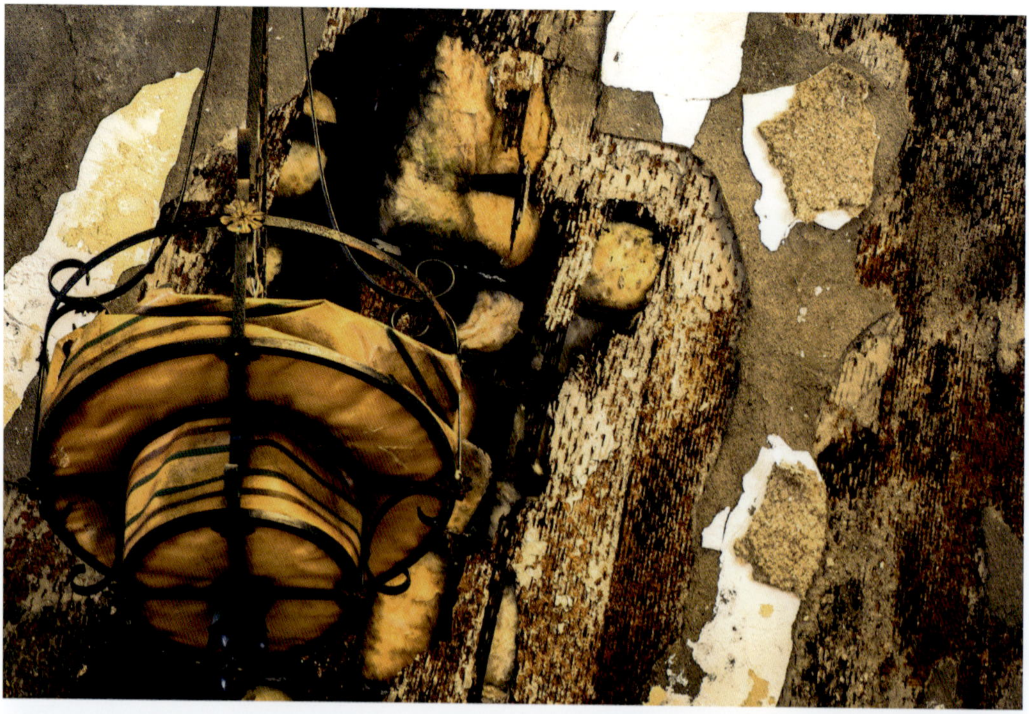

Insulation peeks out of the cracks of ceiling adding to the rusty, braided canvas of decay while the dangling chandelier nearly blends into all of the chaos. *[Photo by Brian Cray]*

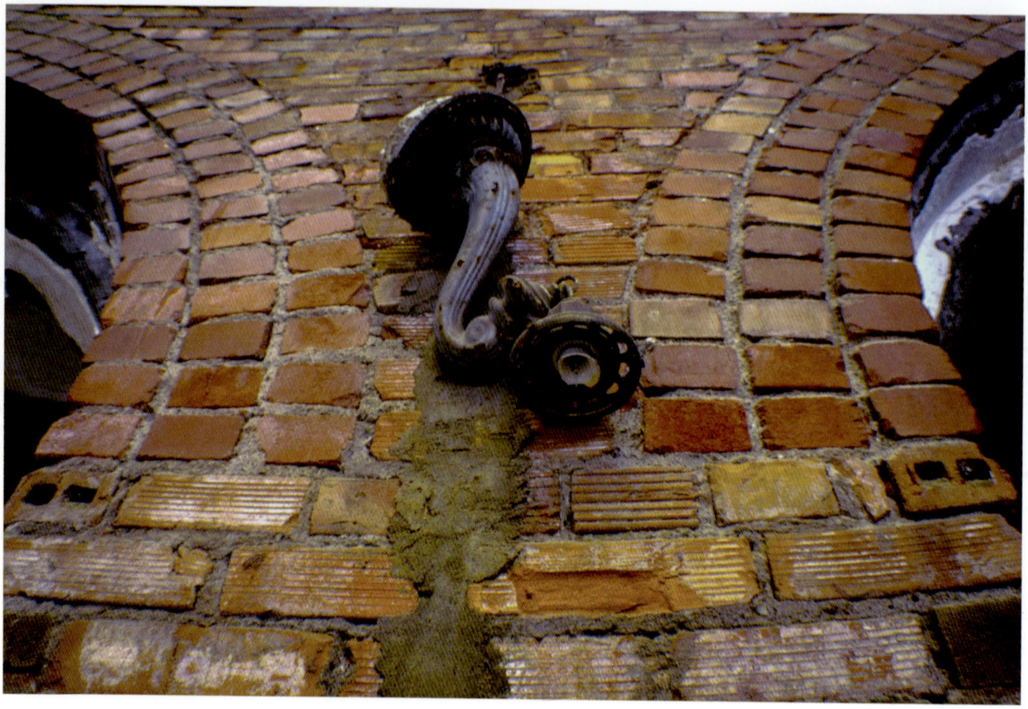

Between the arches of decay light fixtures wilt along her bleeding walls waiting for her bricks to come crumbling down and cover their pain. *[Photo by Brian Cray]*

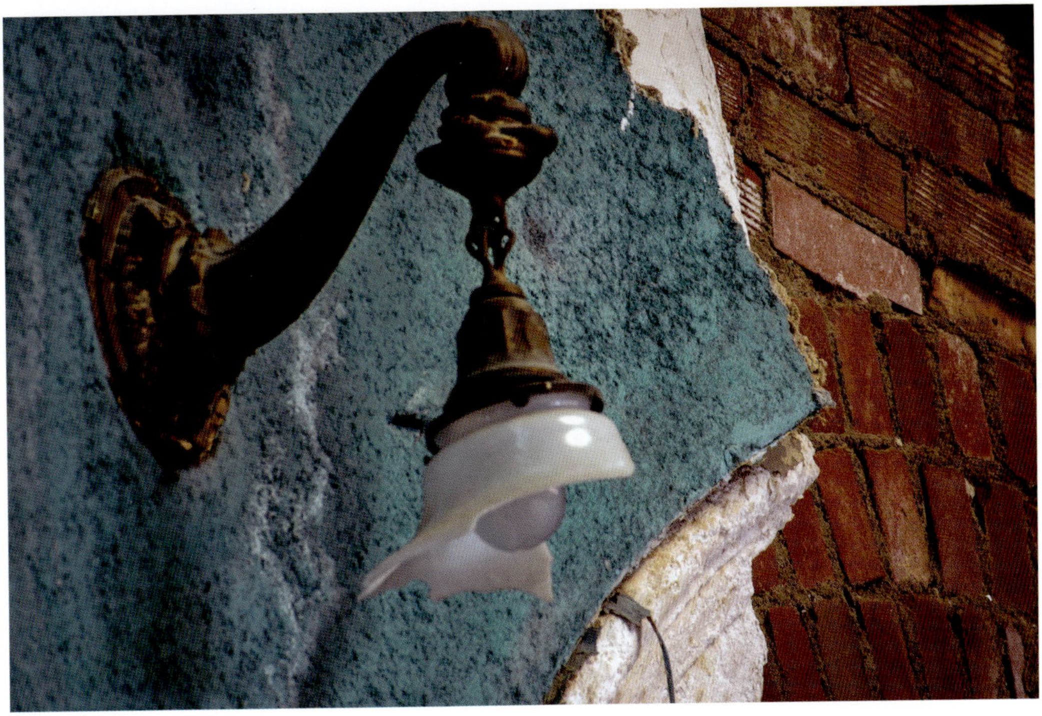

Where the sea meets the red shore the light bulb remains unscathed. Walls slowly come crashing down in pools of plaster and paint and I venture onto Building #3. *[Photo by Brian Cray]*

BUILDING #3 – THE WOMEN'S PULMONARY BUILDING

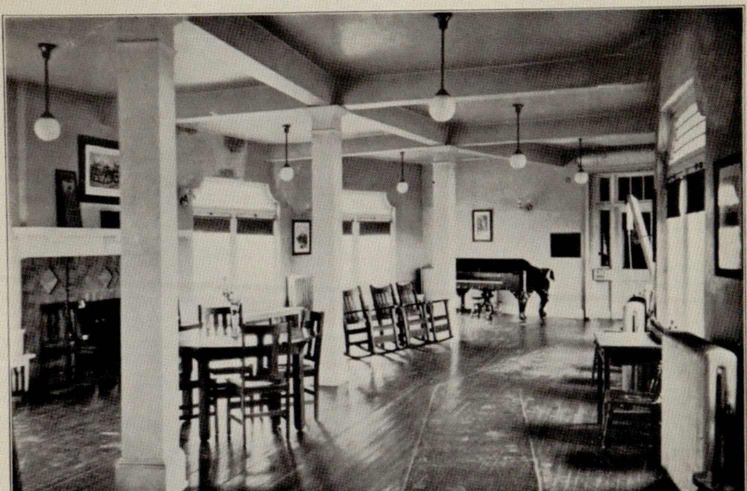

Women' Solarium

Building #3 marks the women's solarium *[Photo by Frank Ruslander, 1920]*

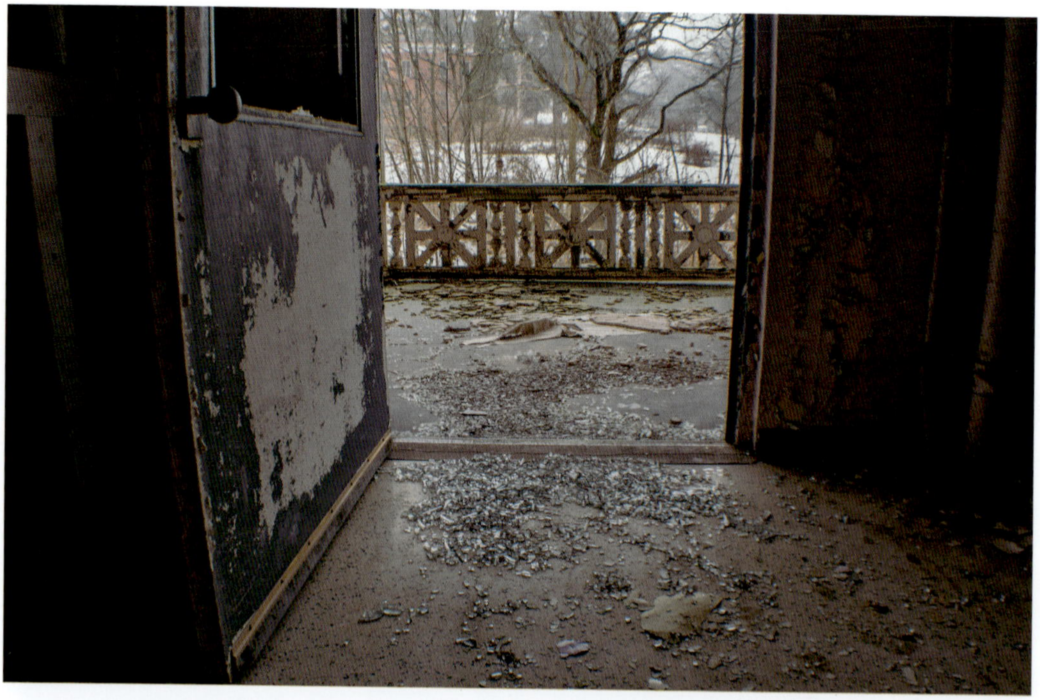

Shattered pain in pulverized bits sprinkles the floor in a mist. If only, if only, she made the list the price would not be the detriment of time. *[Photo by Brian Cray]*

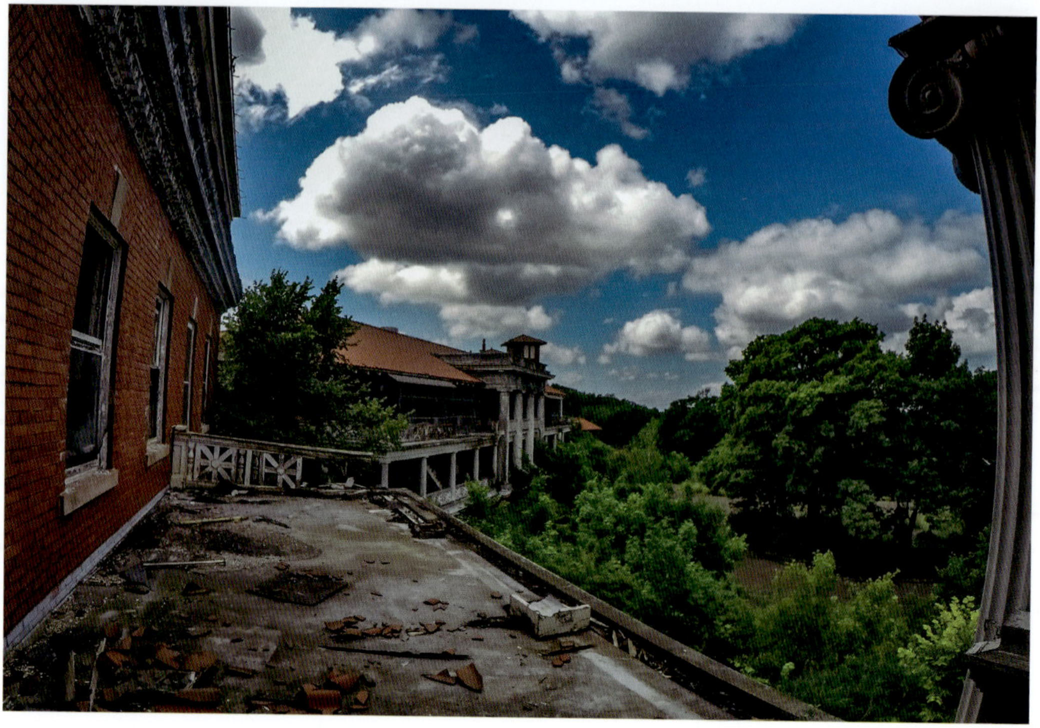

The women's pulmonary ward (Building #3) stretches her ruins across from the main building as I stand on an exposed pavilion void of any balustrade. *[Photo by Brian Cray]*

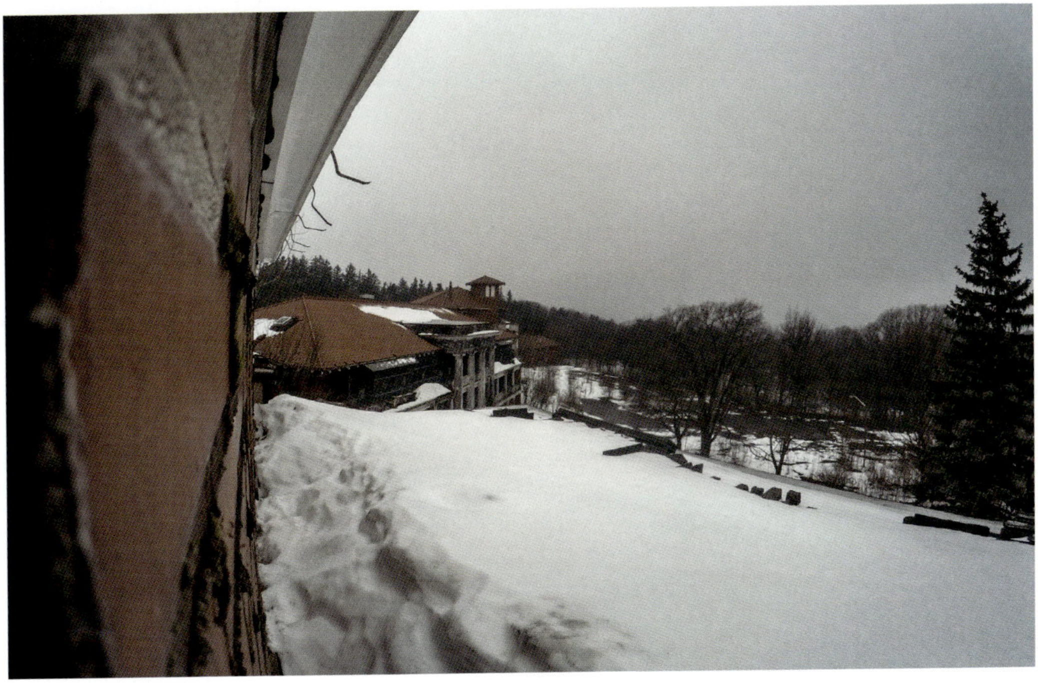

I stand on a white blanket, two years later, looking out at the same edifice slowly crumbling away. With each scream of wind, gentle caress of rain and snow, brings a suffocation of life, but no one can hear her pained silence. *[Photo by Brian Cray]*

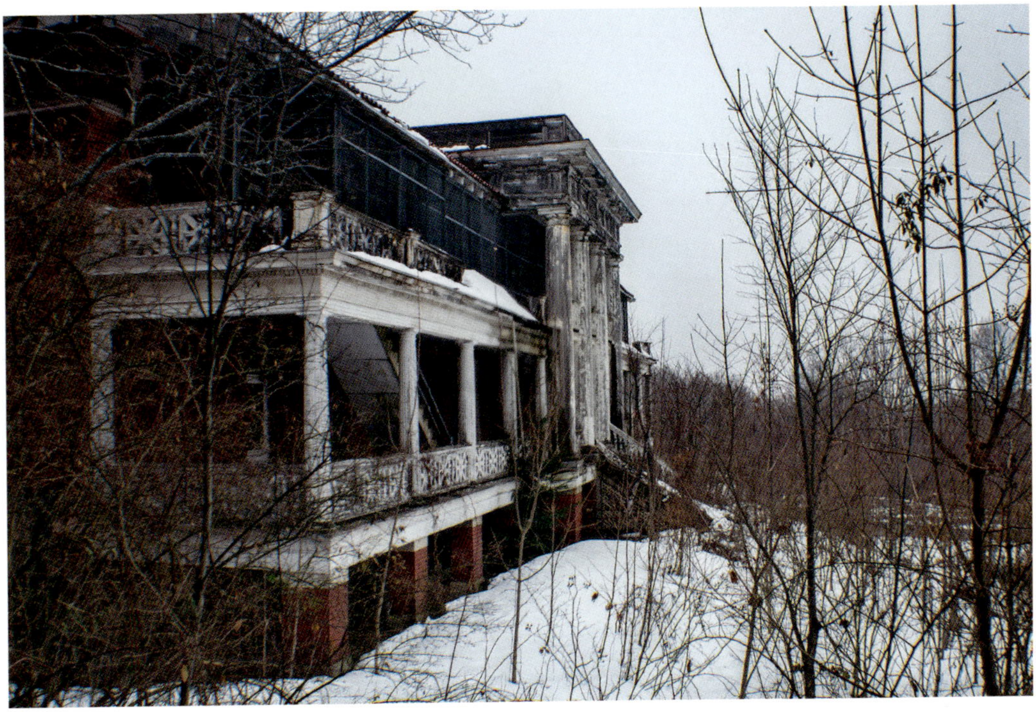

Tuscan Doric Columns guard the façade like a raincoat, but Mother Nature always breaks in with time. *[Photo by Brian Cray]*

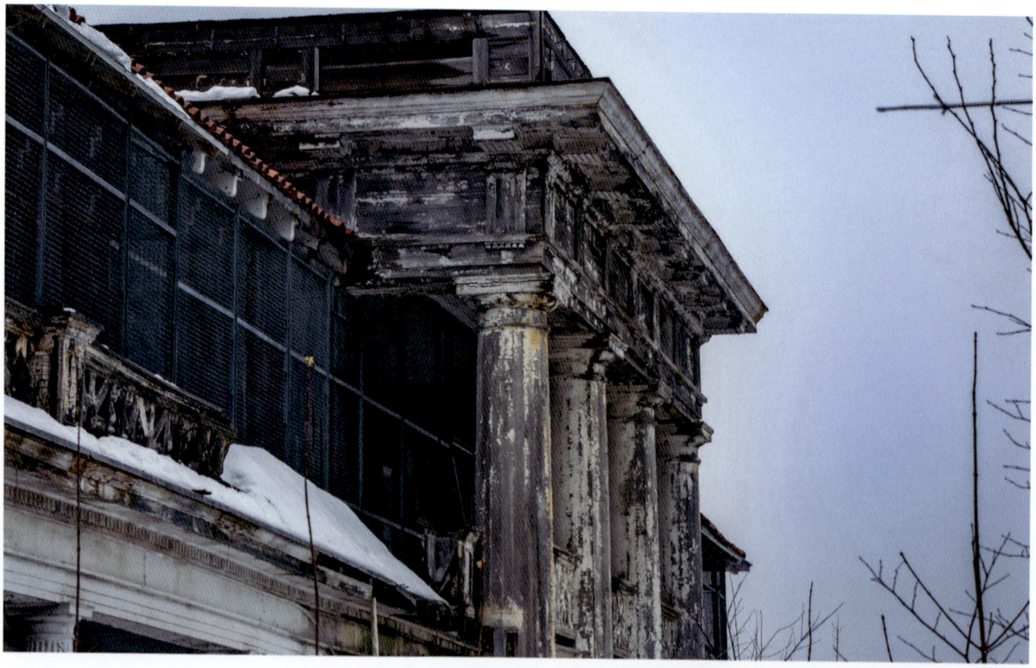

As I zoom in on my camera, I can see the rapid decay melting away the paint of each column to its base like snow disappearing in the midst of sun. Not even the best architectural conservationist can raise these walls from the dead. *[Photo by Brian Cray]*

BUILDING #7

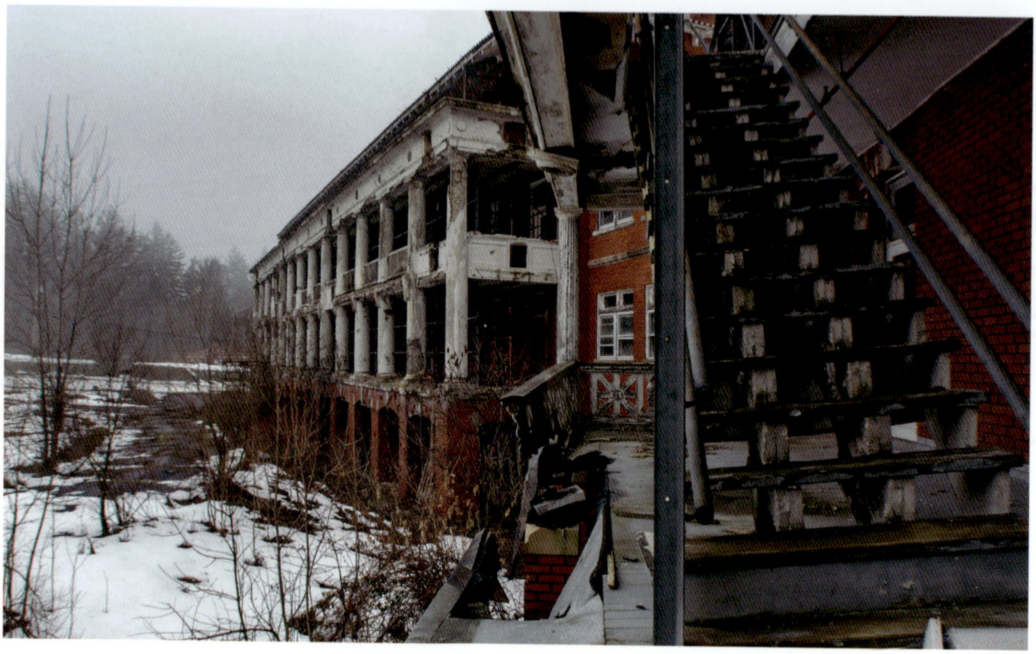

Beyond this stairwell to the women's pulmonary ward rests Building #7, which sits next to Peck Hill Road. I wander quickly and cautiously about the verandas for an incognito presence, hiding behind the emulsion of grays and whites suffocating the sky. *[Photo by Brian Cray]*

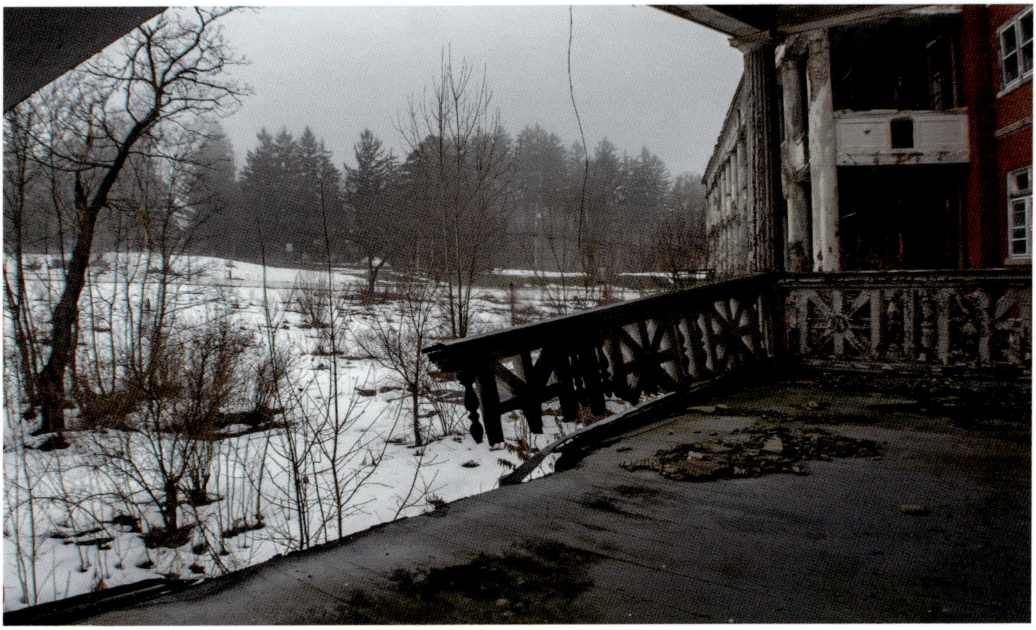

Above: As I look out off the far pavilion of Building #3, I see arson damage that consumed another wooden balustrade. I hear cars approaching in the distance, so I zip in through a French Door and tiptoe back inside to look at her floundering in a war with time. *[Photo by Brian Cray]*

Below left: Empty rooms all paint the same sadness and not even salt can cauterize her wounds. I try to forget the present as I glare into her crystal ball, but I imagine a past just as troubling, full of sickness and undying misery. I could be wrong. *[Photo by Brian Cray]*

Below right: It's hard for me to picture happiness in a time of despair especially when darkness infects the air. I crawl back towards the center of the campus, and wait for the calm of the storm to wander more. *[Photo by Brian Cray]*

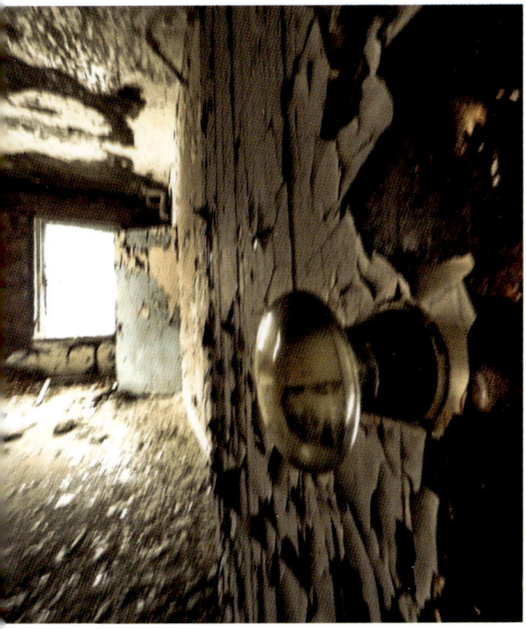

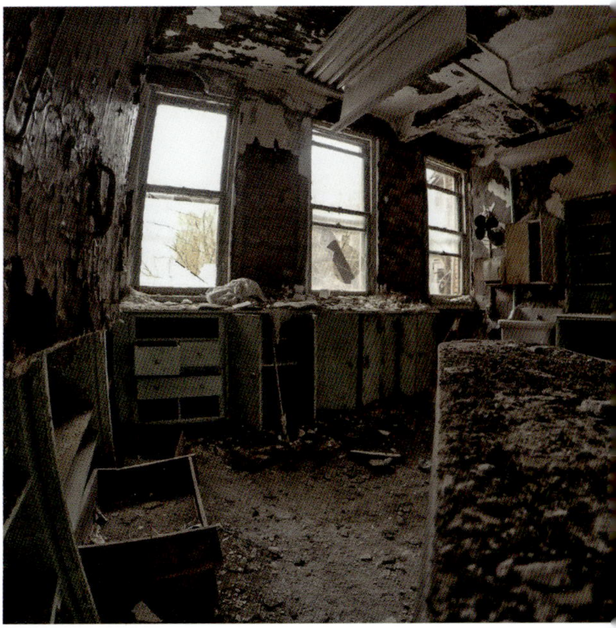

BUILDING #44

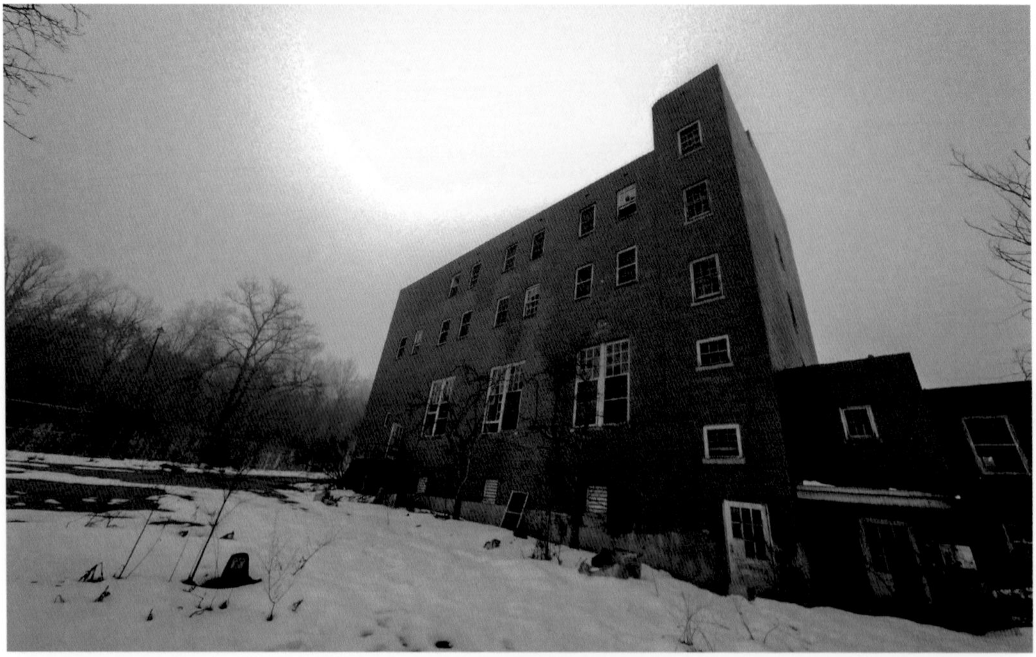

This is Building #44 where the auditorium, operating suite and clinic once operated. Now it's just a shell of the past. *[Photo by Brian Cray]*

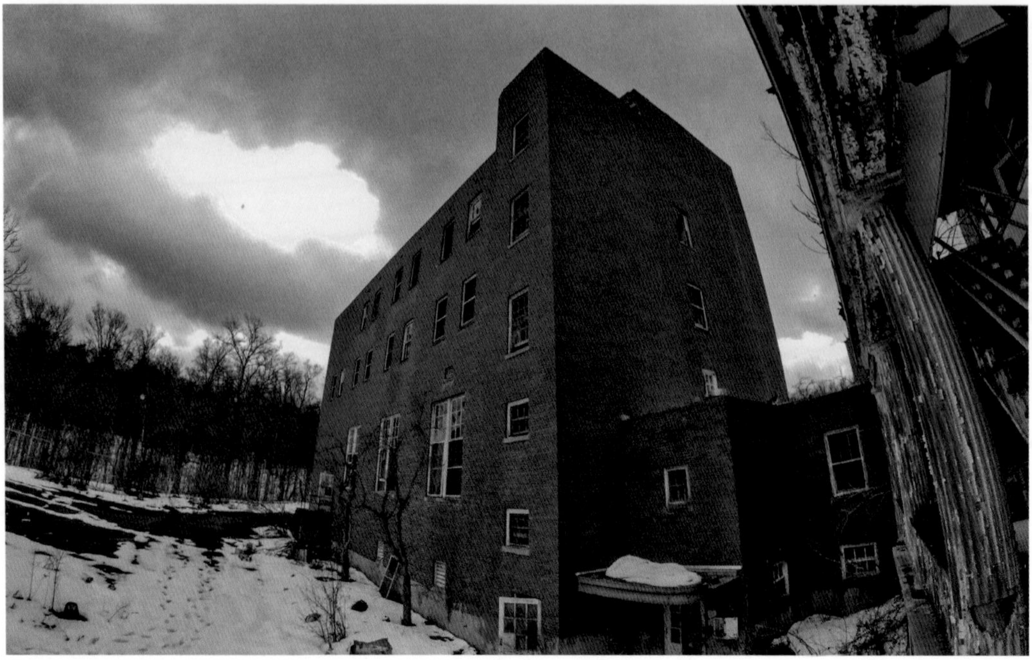

She sits in this cold-mountain town, full of snow, and history. Something about her presence intoxicates me. Maybe it's her lacerated walls, bleeding crimson beneath the daunting sky, her broken windows or crooked screens. *[Photo by Brian Cray]*

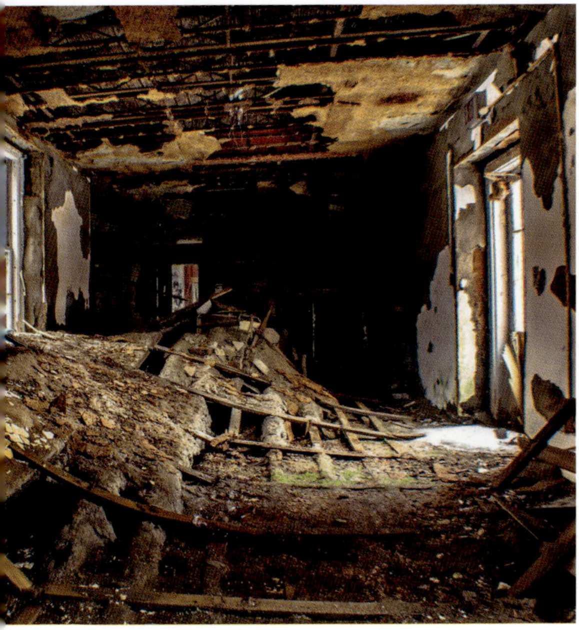

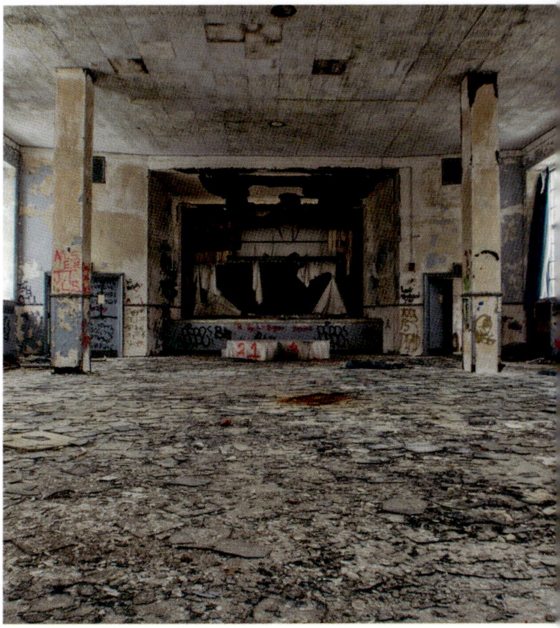

Above left: I stand on swelling floors and cracked boards of chewed debris. I hear a subtle drip disguised as an innocuous melody, but beneath its innocence is the product of decay. *[Photo by Brian Cray]*

Above right: I scramble over ruins and squeeze into the auditorium. It looks like the scene from a horror film as tiles slip under my feet as I walk closer to the podium. *[Photo by Brian Cray]*

Below: Light fixtures suspended from rusted chains wait for an audience to appear. But the only sonorous sounds are a product of wind, the kerplunk of tiles and raindrops or footsteps of trespassers wandering her stage. *[Photo by Brian Cray]*

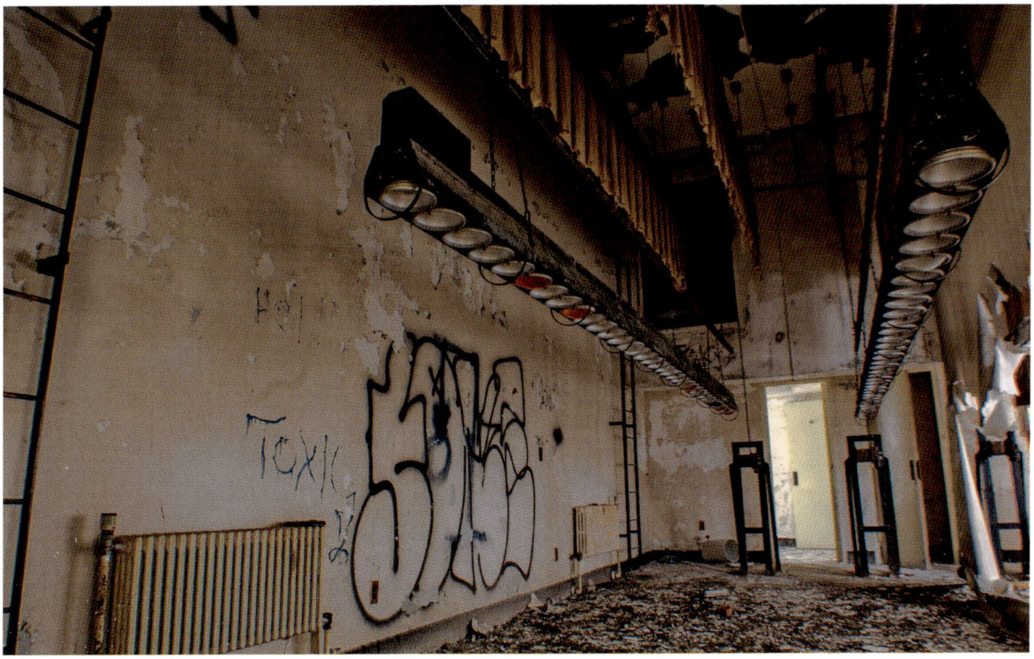

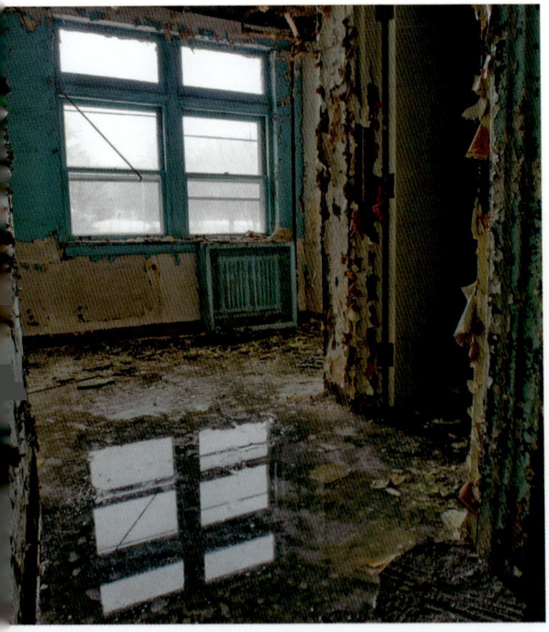

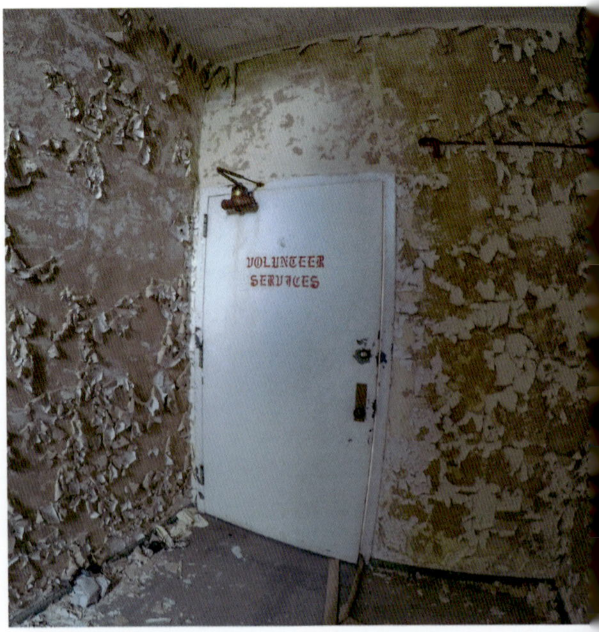

Above left: I wander up a level and watch as frozen memories drown the floor in an ice rink of decay. But puddles of springtime will only open more scars to the ground floor auditorium once her ceiling caves. *[Photo by Brian Cray]*

Above right: Peeling walls flake like a skin disease, but the door to "Volunteer Services" is unaffected by this plague…for now anyway! *[Photo by Brian Cray]*

Below: Step over the discarded tiles as loose debris crunches and clouds the air with stale smoke of decay. *[Photo by Brian Cray]*

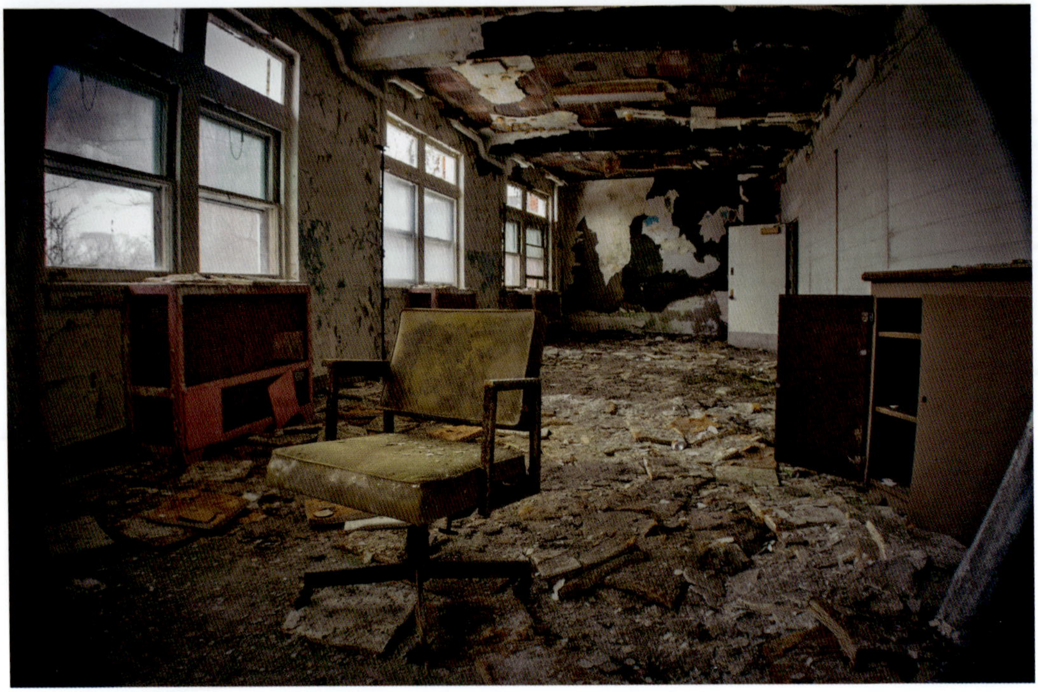

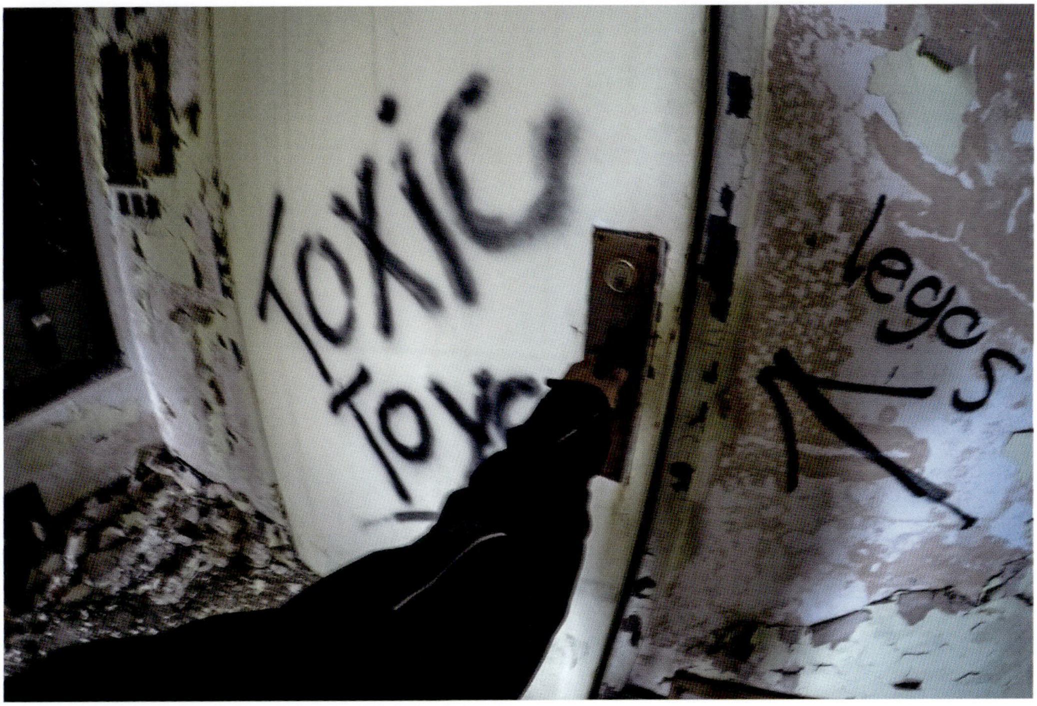

Toxic Toys for girls and boys. PROCEED! *[Photo by Brian Cray]*

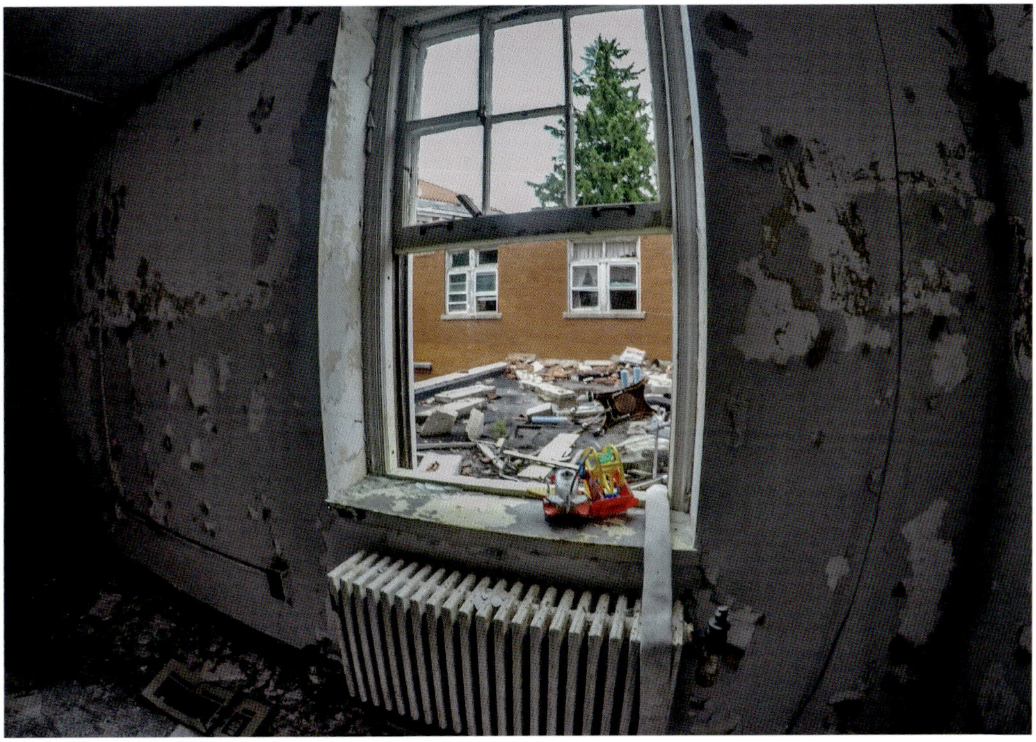

As I wander further, I stand in her shadows of perishing remains. I glare out at the few toys that wait on the windowsill for a child to play with them, but their lives as toys died long ago. *[Photo by Brian Cray]*

BUILDING #2 – THE MEN'S PULMONARY WARD

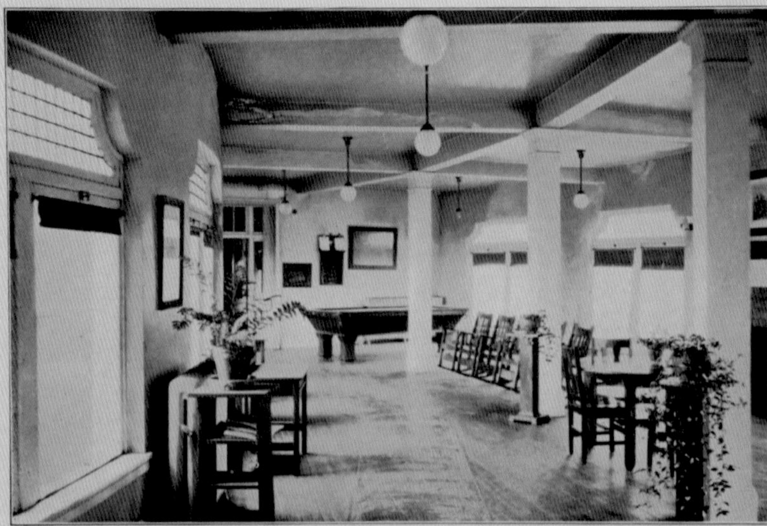

Men's Solarium or Recreation Room

[Photo by Frank Ruslander, 1920]

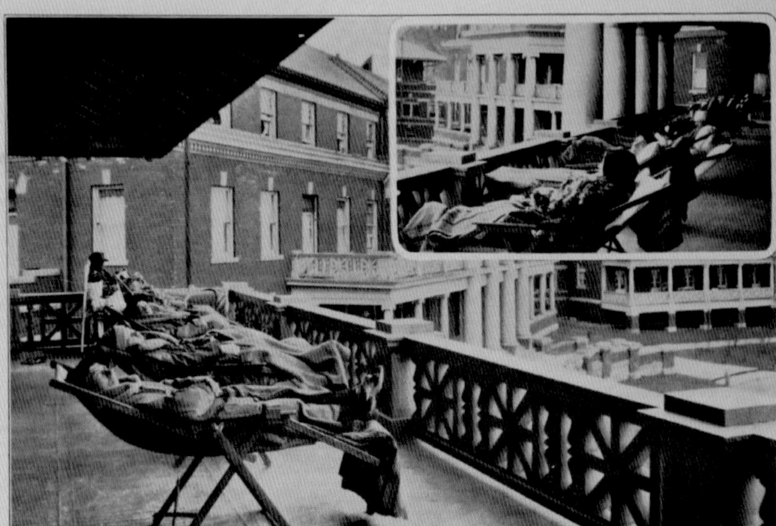

Pulmonary Patients taking Air Cure
The Patients lie in these Chairs Six Hours a Day, Winter and Summer

[Photo by Frank Ruslander, 1920]

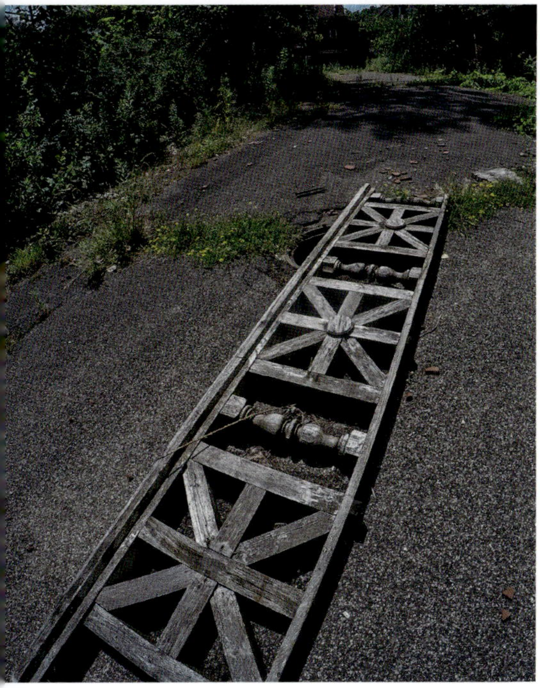

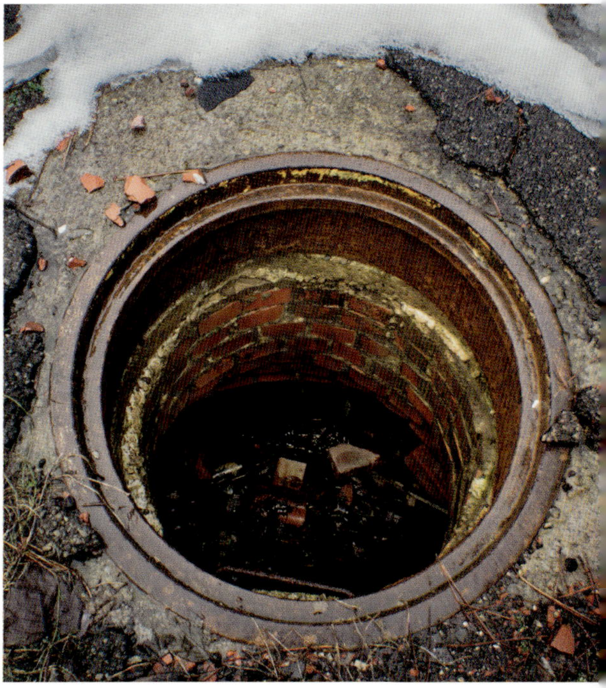

Above left: A section of wooden balustrade, once covered in white paint, lies amidst the cracked asphalt of her ruins. *[Photo by Brian Cray]*

Above right: As I look at the eye in the ground, I see chunks of brick, glass beer bottles, and the darkest water. The contamination from the ruins seeps slowly into the open voids of earth like melting snow. *[Photo by Brian Cray]*

Below: Lush forest piles on for miles behind decaying edifices. Beneath the clouds and blue sky, the Great Lakes ripple in the distance, home to the most shipwrecks per square mile (Guerrieri, 2018). *[Photo by Brian Cray]*

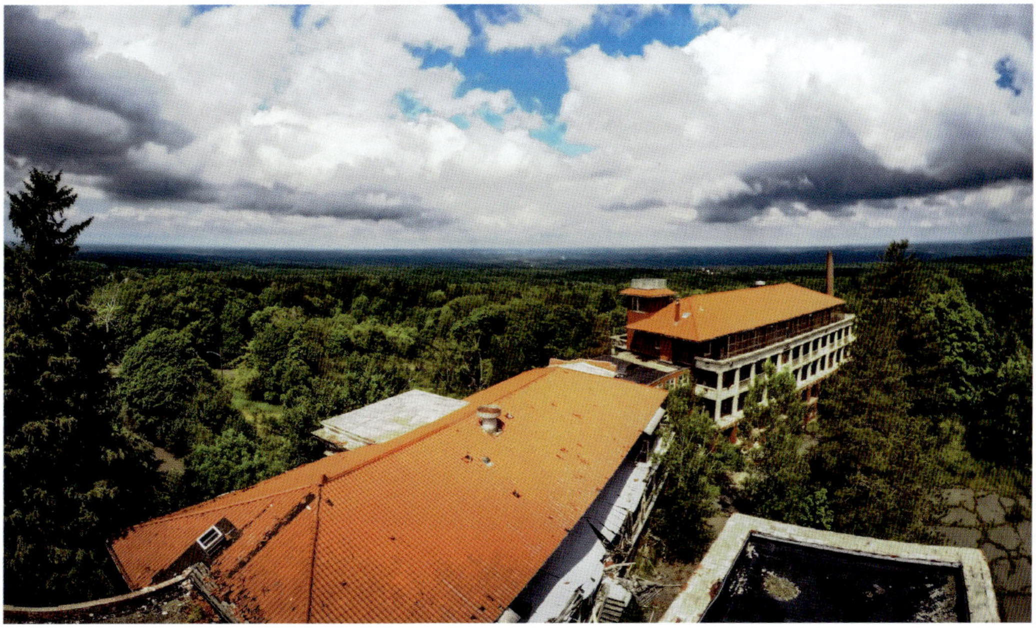

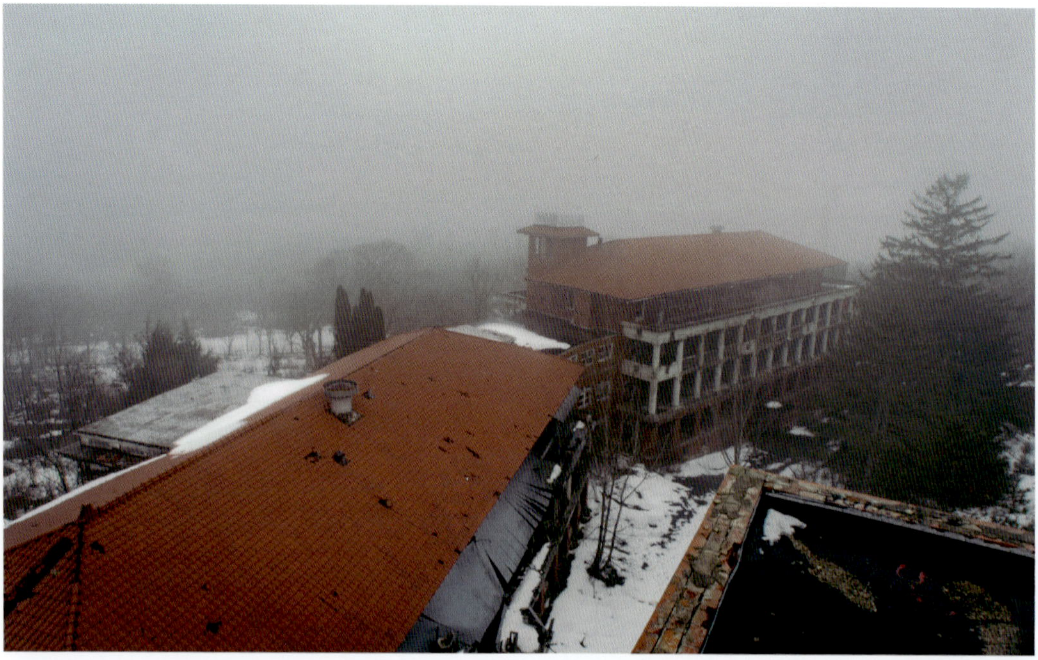

Two years later I snap a flick of the same view from the rooftop of Building #44. Winter fog and mist emits an eerie feeling across the campus. The depressing winter months definitely affected the sun cure. *[Photo by Brian Cray]*

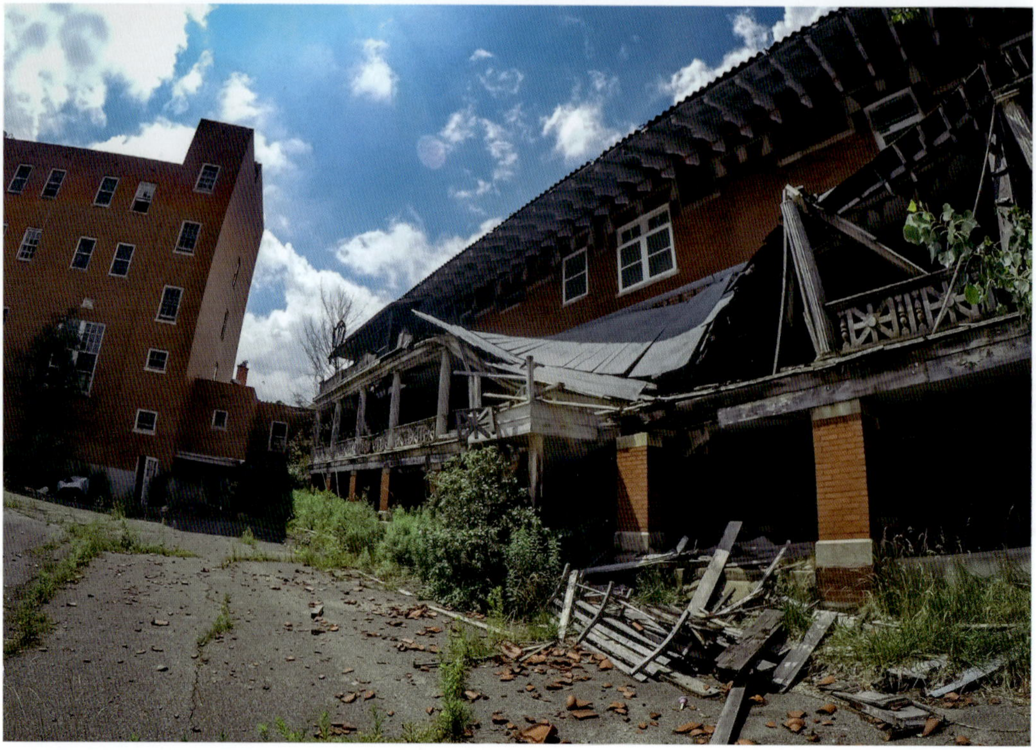

Tumbled bits of wood and brick decorate the parking lot as the awning to Building #2 slumps to the floor of the veranda. *[Photo by Brian Cray]*

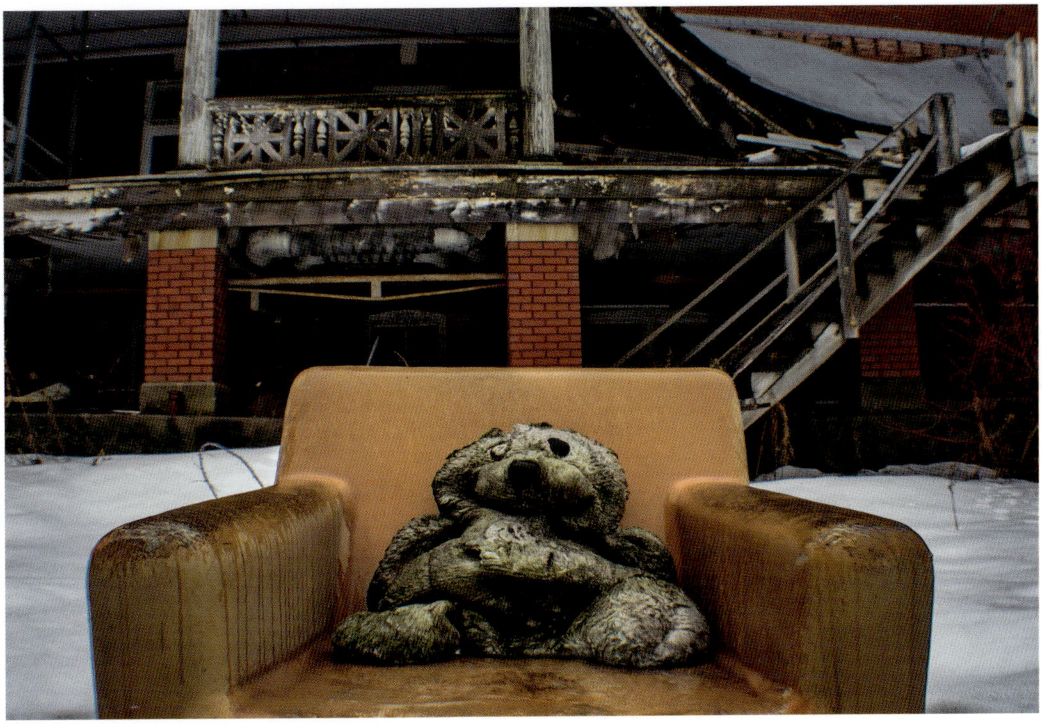

Teddy sits there in a deep stare with ruffled fur and without a care. *[Photo by Brian Cray]*

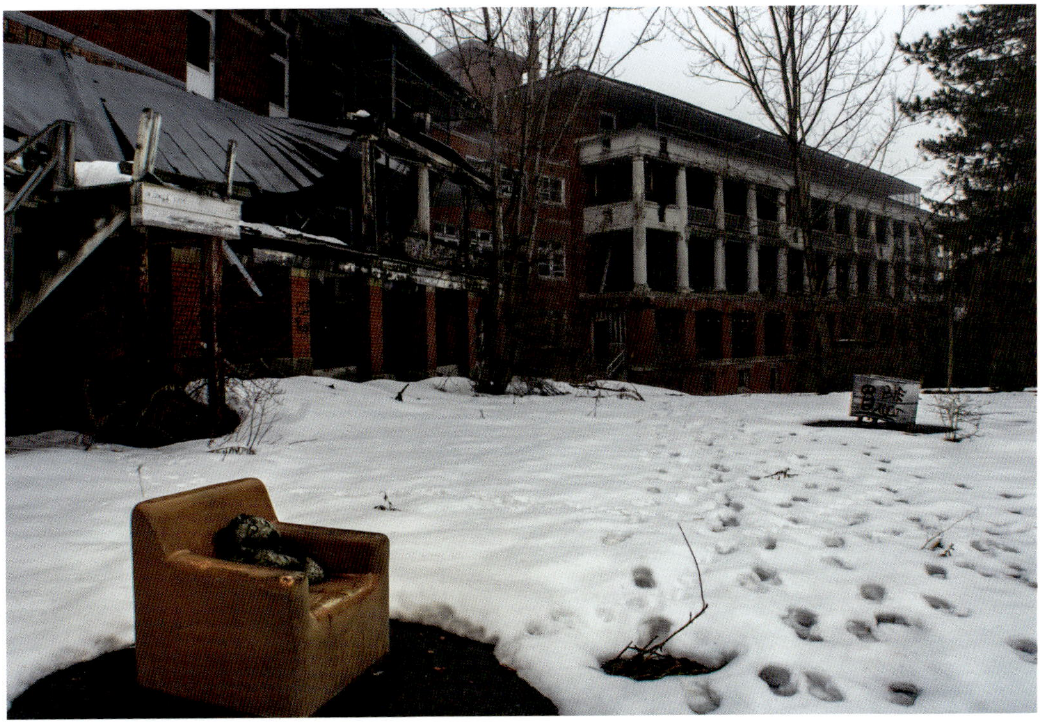

It is doubtful Teddy was a toy from the sanitarium. I did not see this here in 2016 on my first visit so it's more plausible that a vandal left him behind. *[Photo by Brian Cray]*

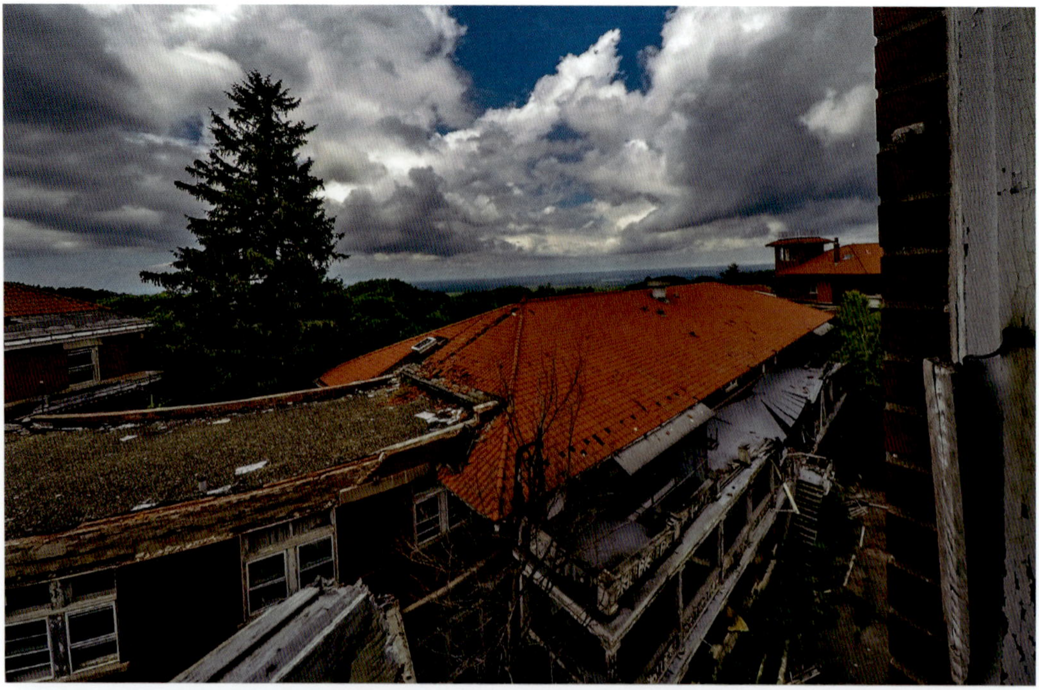

As I lean out the splintered window of Building #44, I see a crippled complex. Much like her patients who lived with Consumption she too suffers the incurable decadence of time. *[Photo by Brian Cray]*

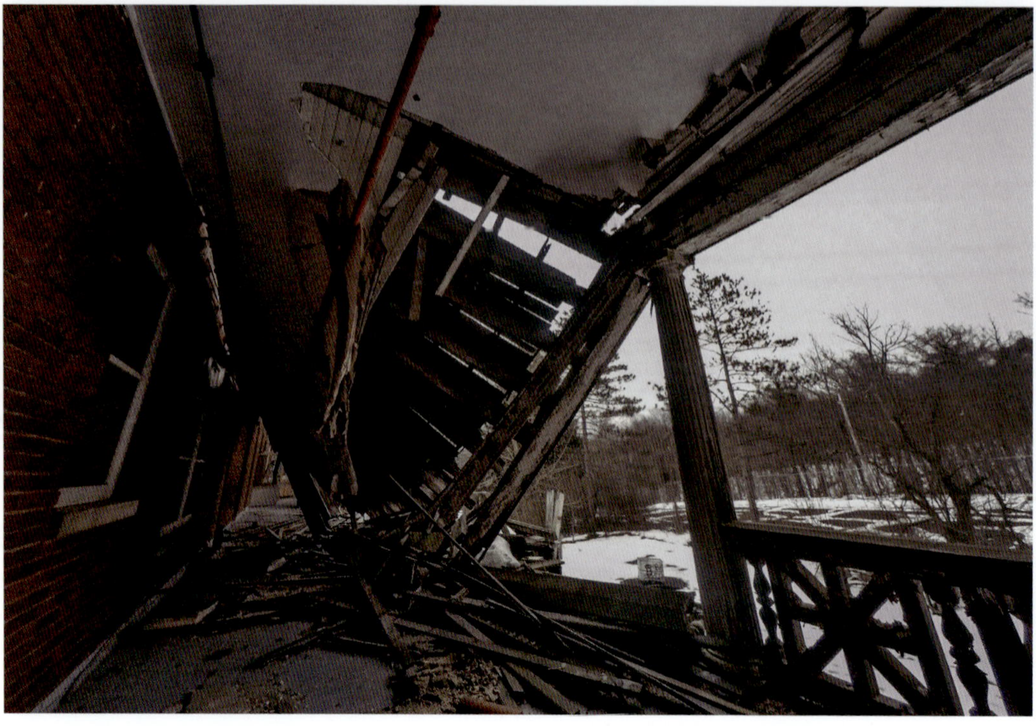

The surreal distortion feeds the illusion of her brick walls caving outwards. But there is no conjuring to her collapsed ceiling sweeping the floor with heaps of wood. *[Photo by Brian Cray]*

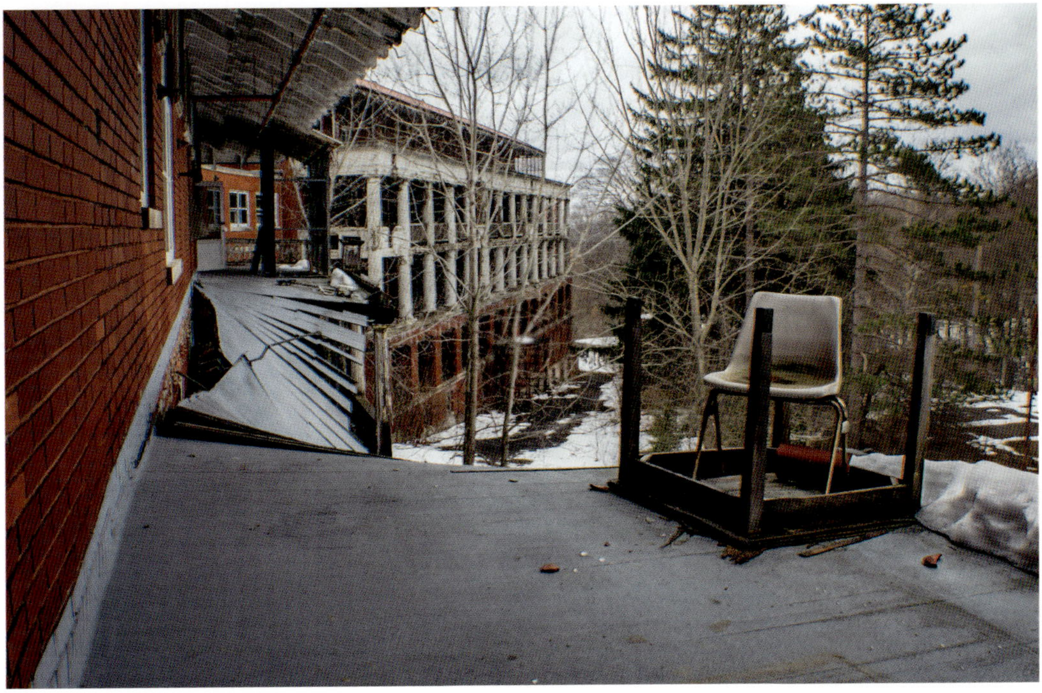

The sun seldom stares through the dreary clouds of winter, but in summer, take cover, the undulating rays can make you queasy. Be sure to not fall through the floor! *[Photo by Brian Cray]*

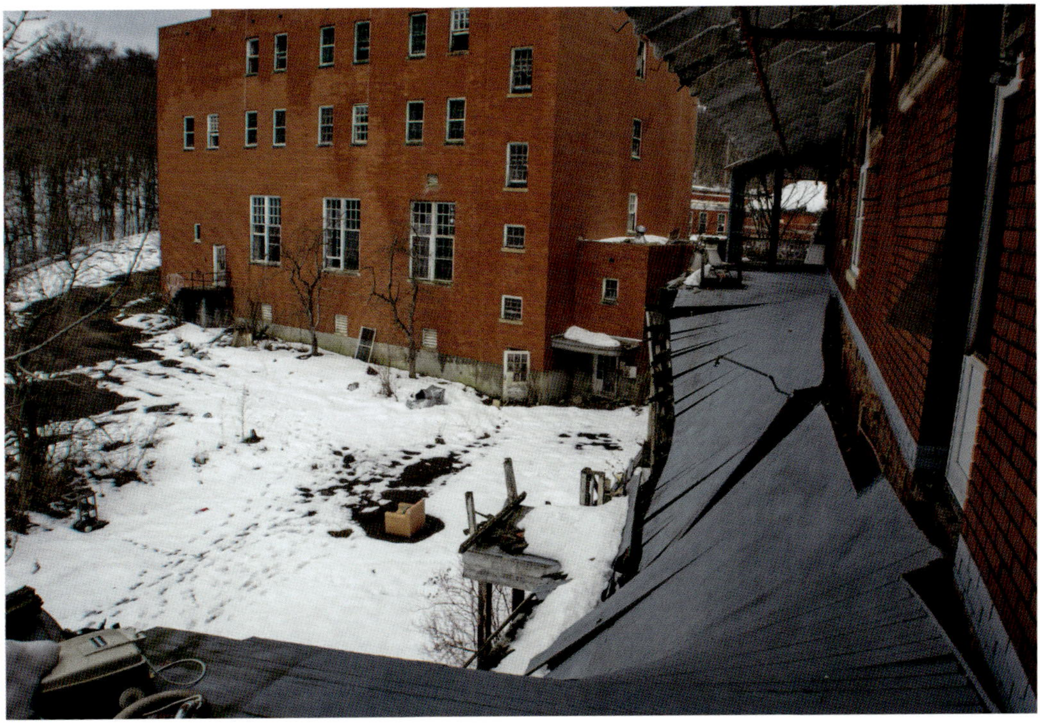

I look across the same veranda standing on the opposite side for a better view at the wrought loggia. She twists and turns like a roller coaster as my toes tremble in trepidation. *[Photo by Brian Cray]*

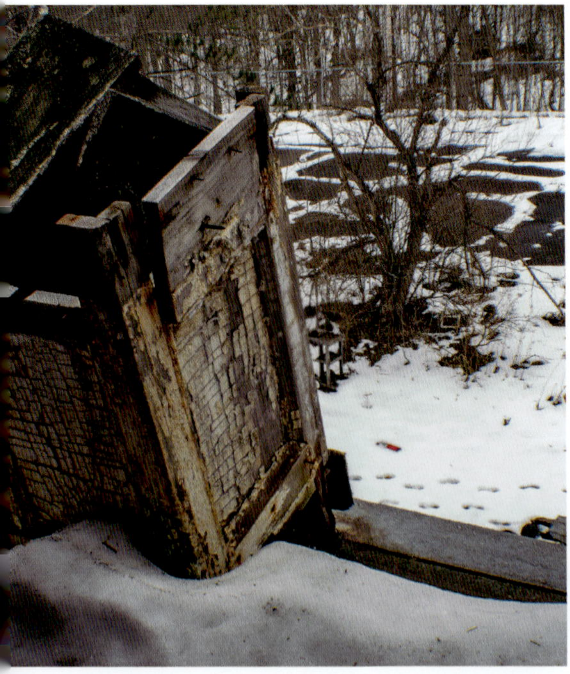

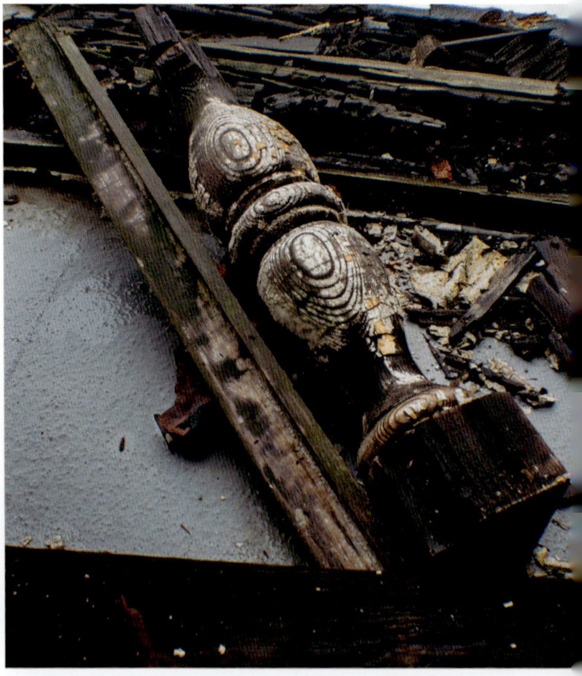

Above left: Wooden column slumps at its base with loose and rusty teeth birthing cavities of decay. *[Photo by Brian Cray]*

Above right: Wood grains bleed through layers of warped decay and fester in a pile of charred ruins. *[Photo by Brian Cray]*

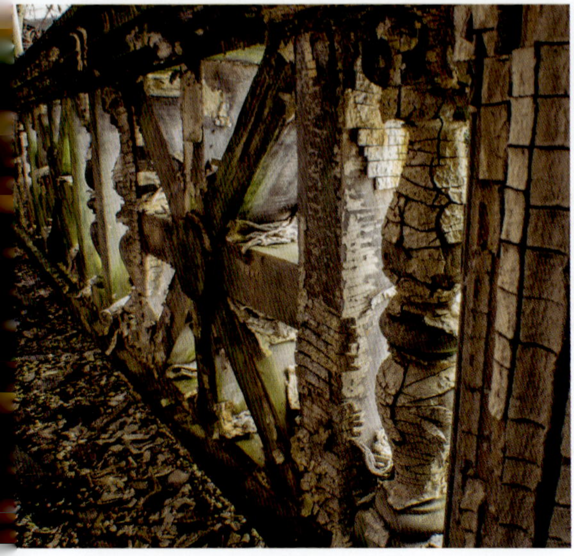

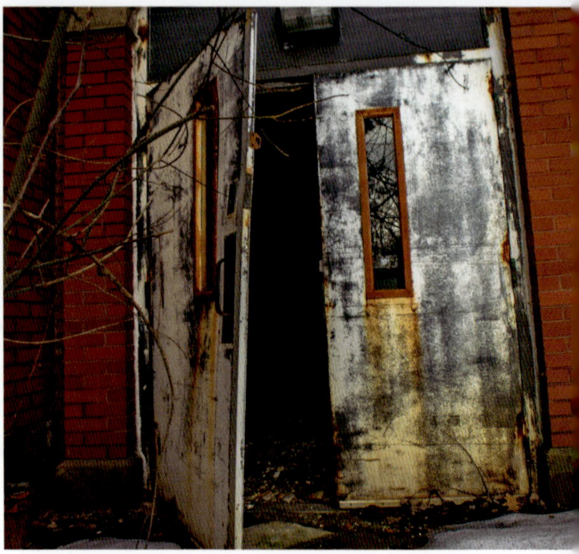

Above left: Leprosy spreads along the wooden banisters like the vines of a Banyan tree bleeding her of life. *[Photo by Brian Cray]*

Above right: Tears of rust stain French Doors and her creaking hinges pierce my ears from the blistering wind. I creep inside and brace myself for what's to come. *[Photo by Brian Cray]*

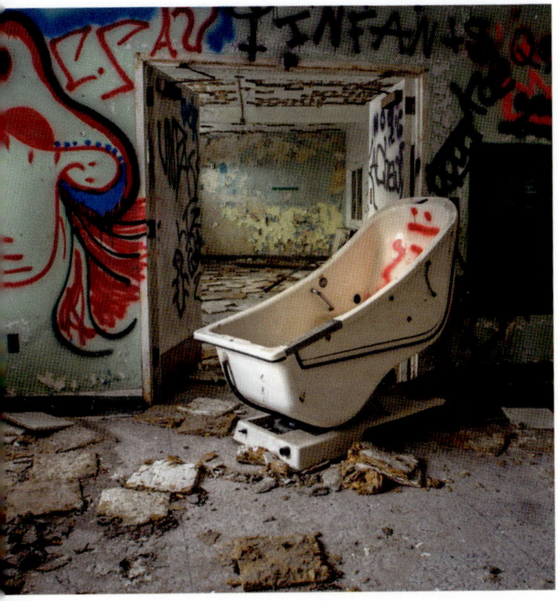

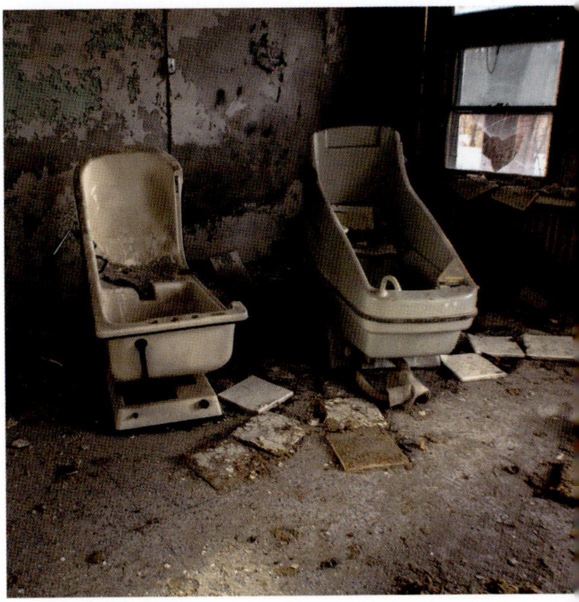

Above left: "Toy" graffiti crowds sage walls behind an old Invacare shower system presumably used to bathe disabled patients from the days of the J. N. Adam Developmental Center. *[Photo by Brian Cray]*

Above right: In total, I witnessed three Invacare shower systems, all fairly intact, with slight signs of decay. *[Photo by Brian Cray]*

Below: I would presume this was expensive equipment for its time as these bath systems nowadays are the upwards of several thousand dollars for both the system and installation. *[Photo by Brian Cray]*

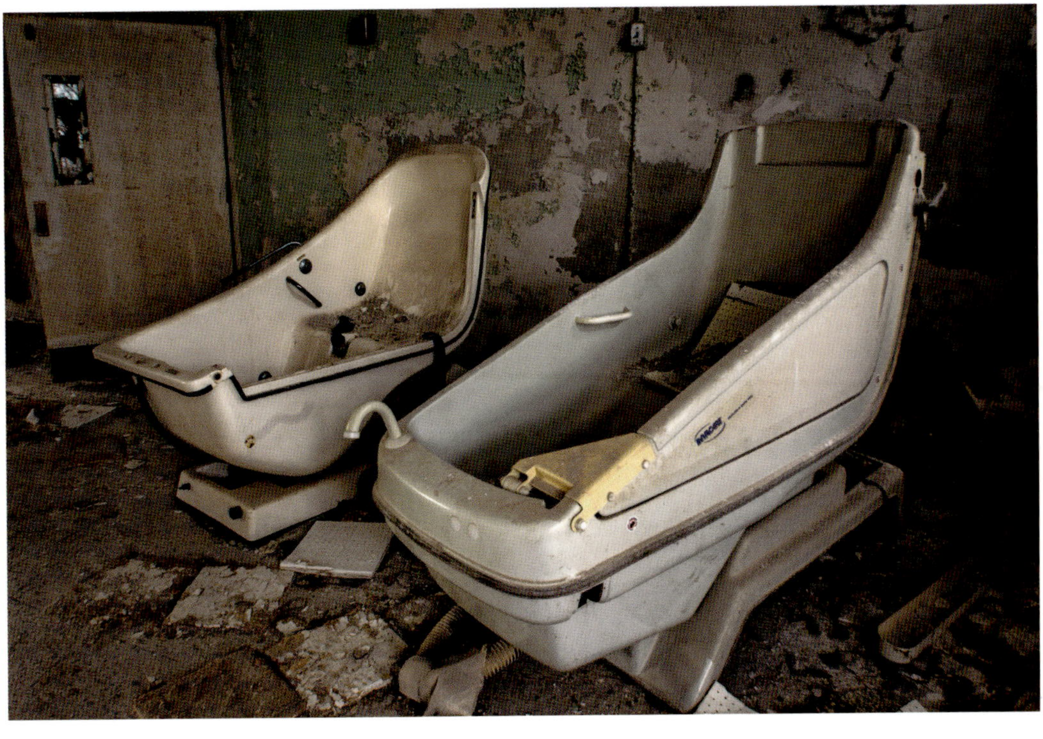

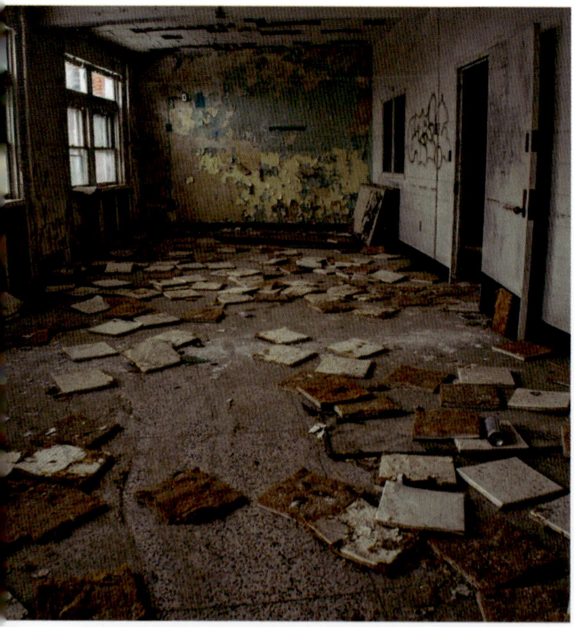

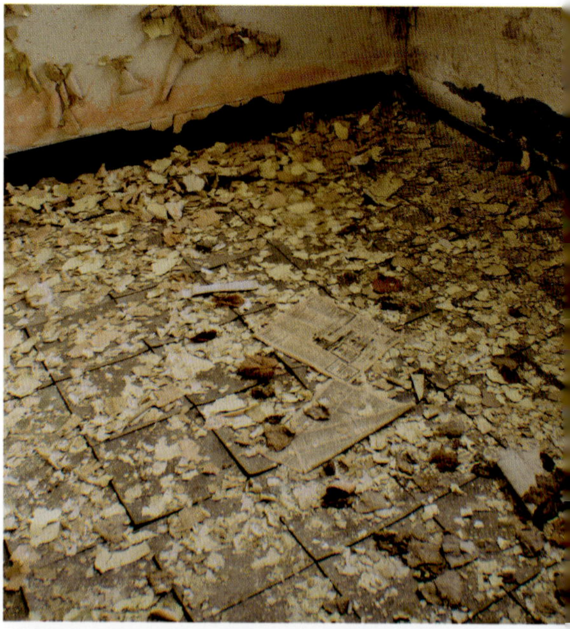

Above left: Tiles from the ceiling drown the floor like patches of shag carpet from the 80s. Her ruins have lived on through many decades. *[Photo by Brian Cray]*

Above right: Chips of lemon-meringue paint crumb the loose tiles of floor and I wonder how many other old newspaper clippings were left behind to be forgotten in her crumbling walls. *[Photo by Brian Cray]*

Below: I haven't seen one of these tube monitors since the early 90s when AOL dialup came on CD's and it took hours to download an MP3. *[Photo by Brian Cray]*

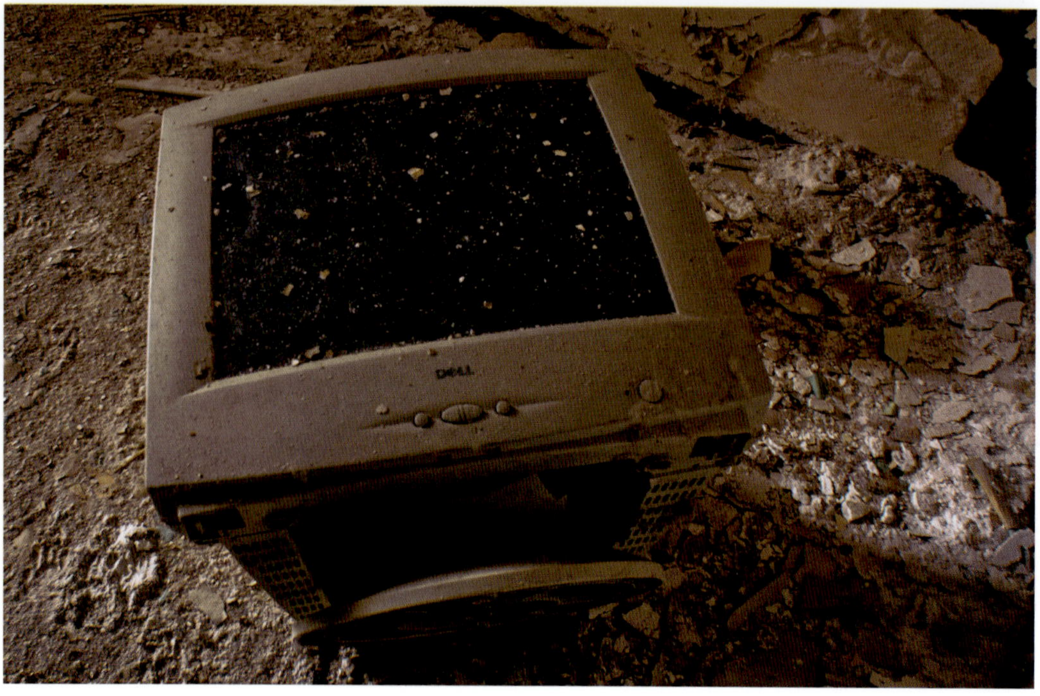

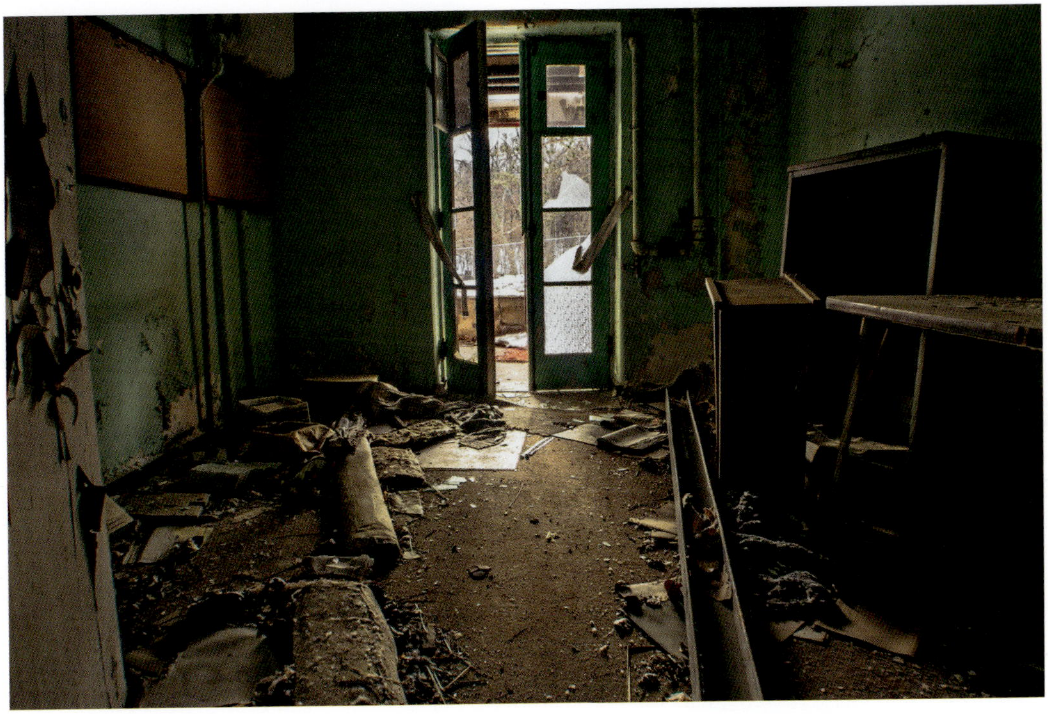

Ambient light shines in through busted, frosted glass unveiling the mystery of what's to come. Slowly my eyes dart to the ruins spread across the floor and I see her predestined fate. *[Photo by Brian Cray]*

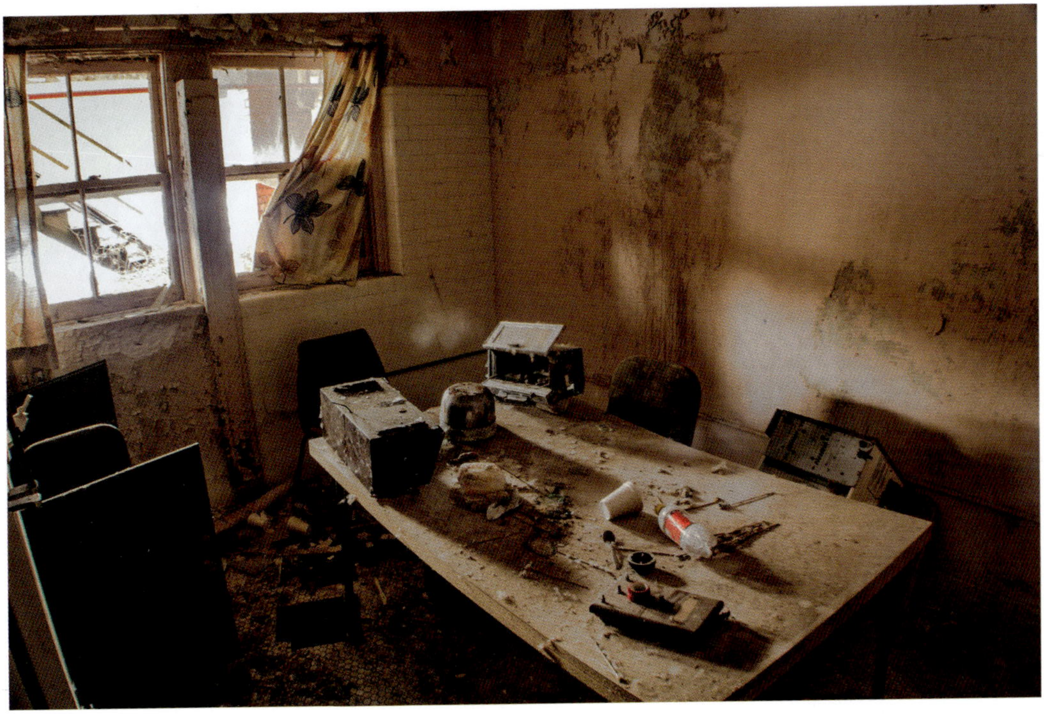

Appliances rot away between the dust and feathers of rapid decay as honeycombs immerge from the flooring. *[Photo by Brian Cray]*

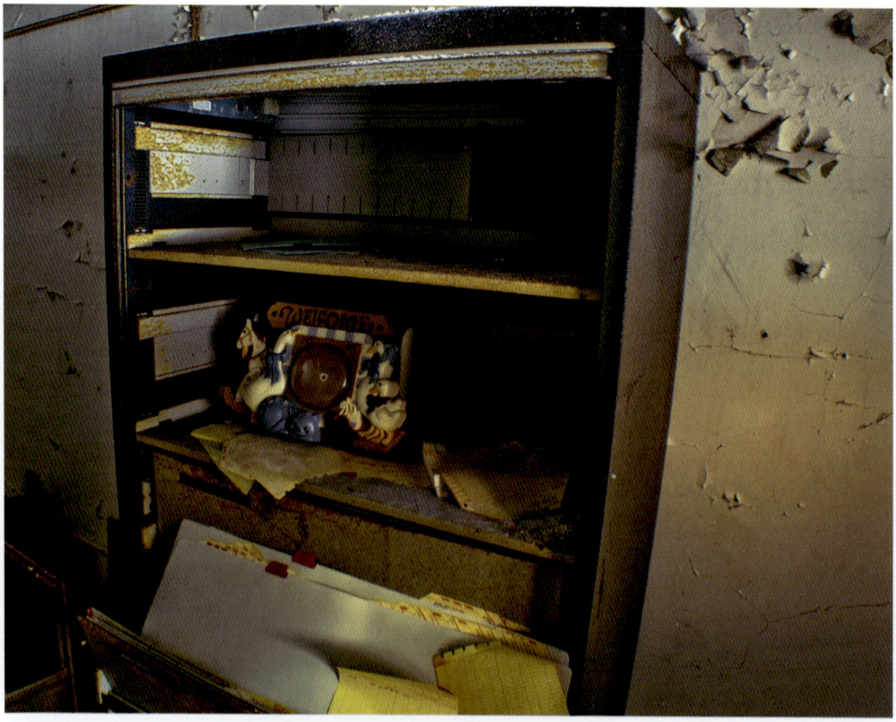

"WELCOME!" This piece reached out to me and grabbed my eyes for it felt too new and unblemished. It did not fit with the rest of the decaying toys and knickknacks or maybe it did? *[Photo by Brian Cray]*

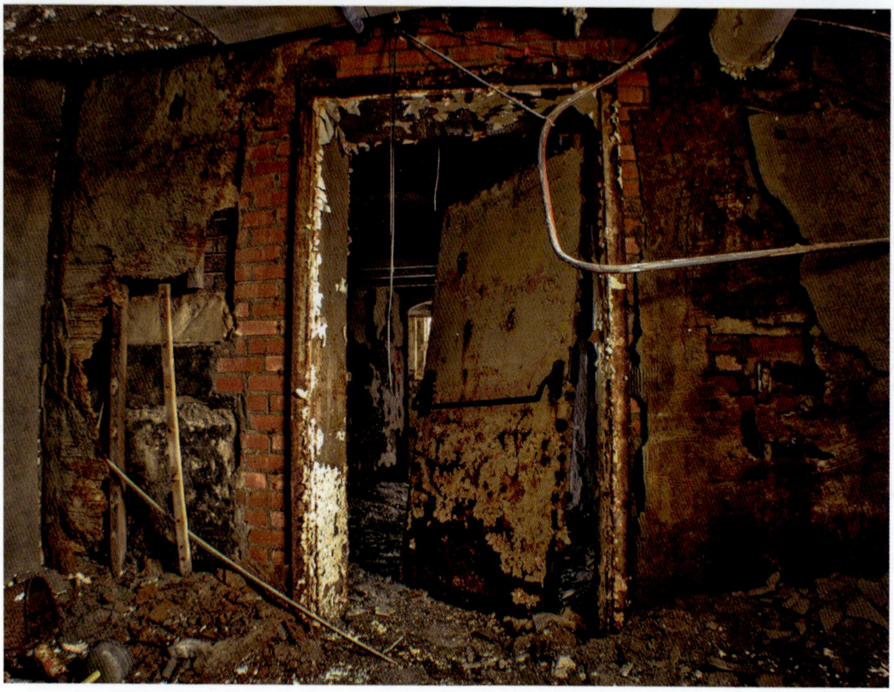

The door slumps, goading me into the next room, amidst earth-shattering mush. I can feel her pressing down on my head or maybe it's just my imagination. *[Photo by Brian Cray]*

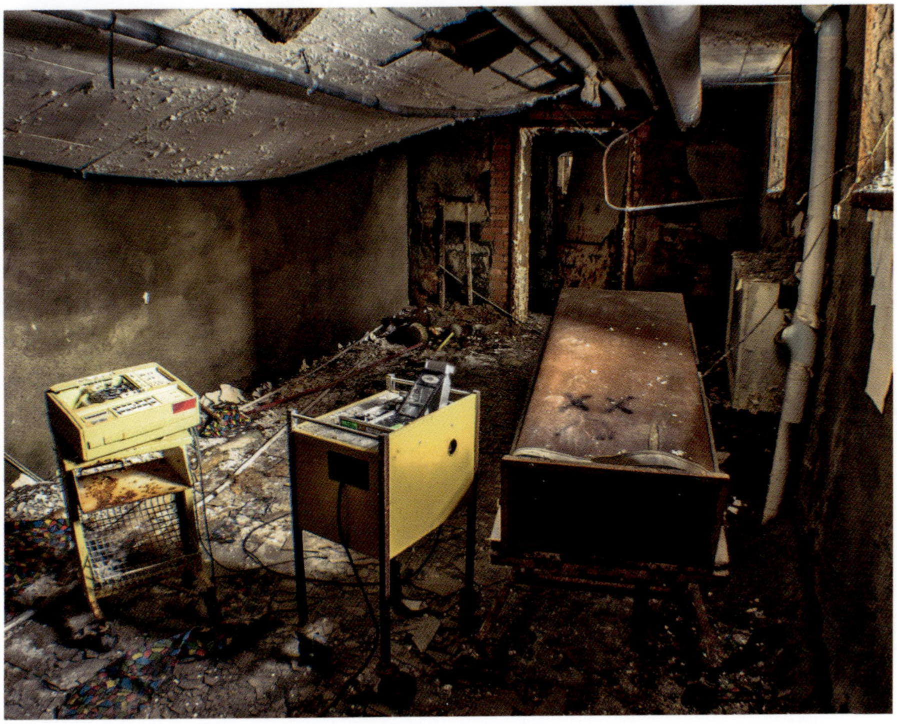

I can only wonder what tests physicians administered on their patients with these machines. But with all the commotion, I cannot take my eyes off her bulging ceiling and cataclysmic cries. *[Photo by Brian Cray]*

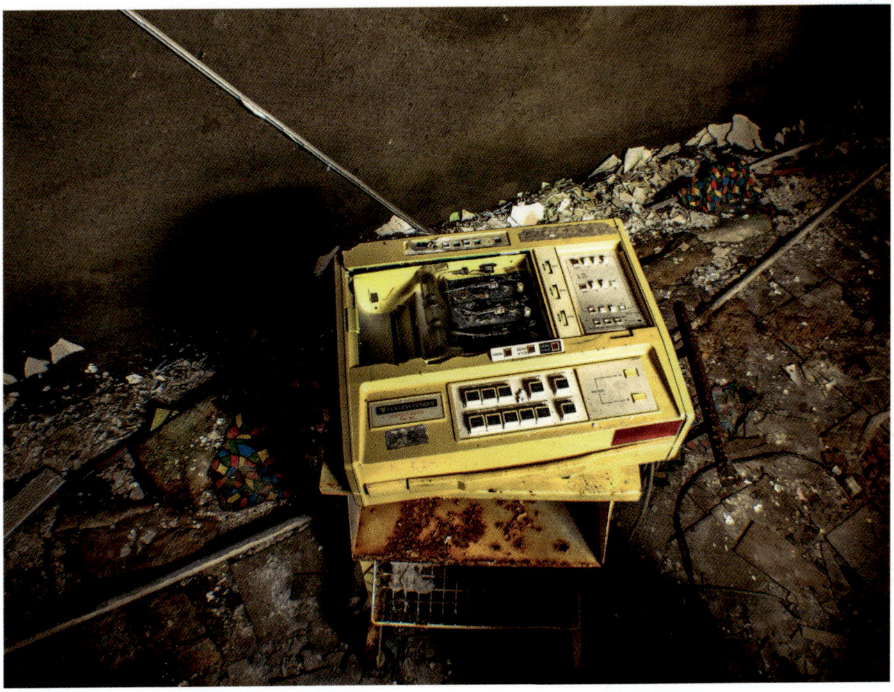

A shadow engulfs the machine like the presence of death, and I look down to read the label, "Fukuda Denshi Cardio Auto FD-36" *[Photo by Brian Cray]*

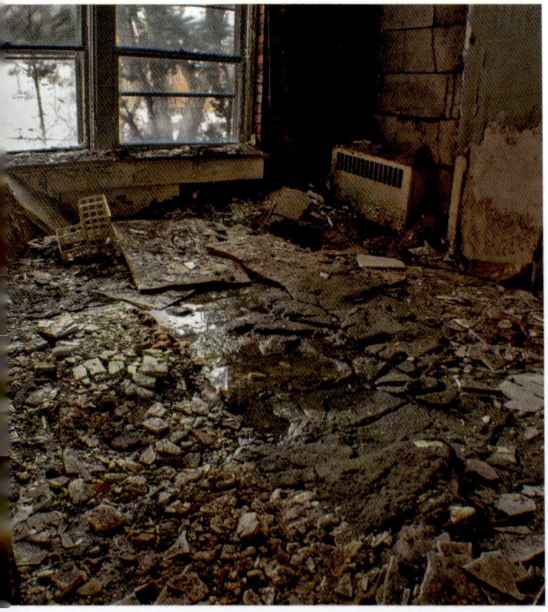

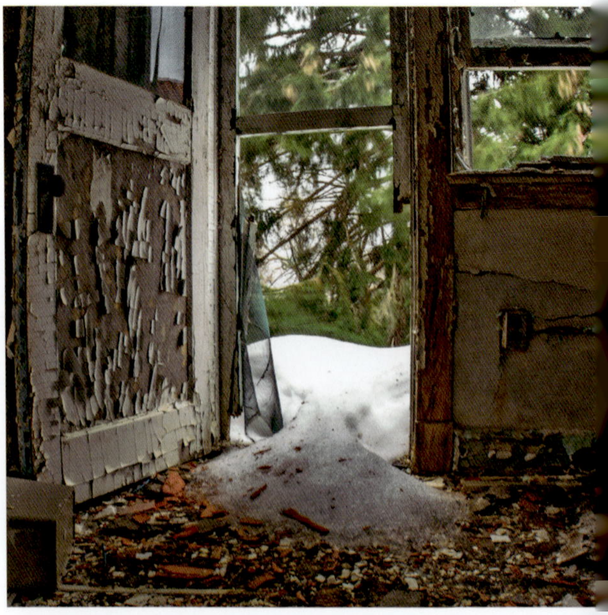

Above left: Each room I wander past looks the same as the one before a landfill of forgotten memories and defunct medical practices. *[Photo by Brian Cray]*

Above right: Majestic beauty comes in many forms and through many storms. *[Photo by Brian Cray]*

Below: All of the furniture that survived the years rests outside. Take a seat. Imagine her past and wander through her memories. *[Photo by Brian Cray]*

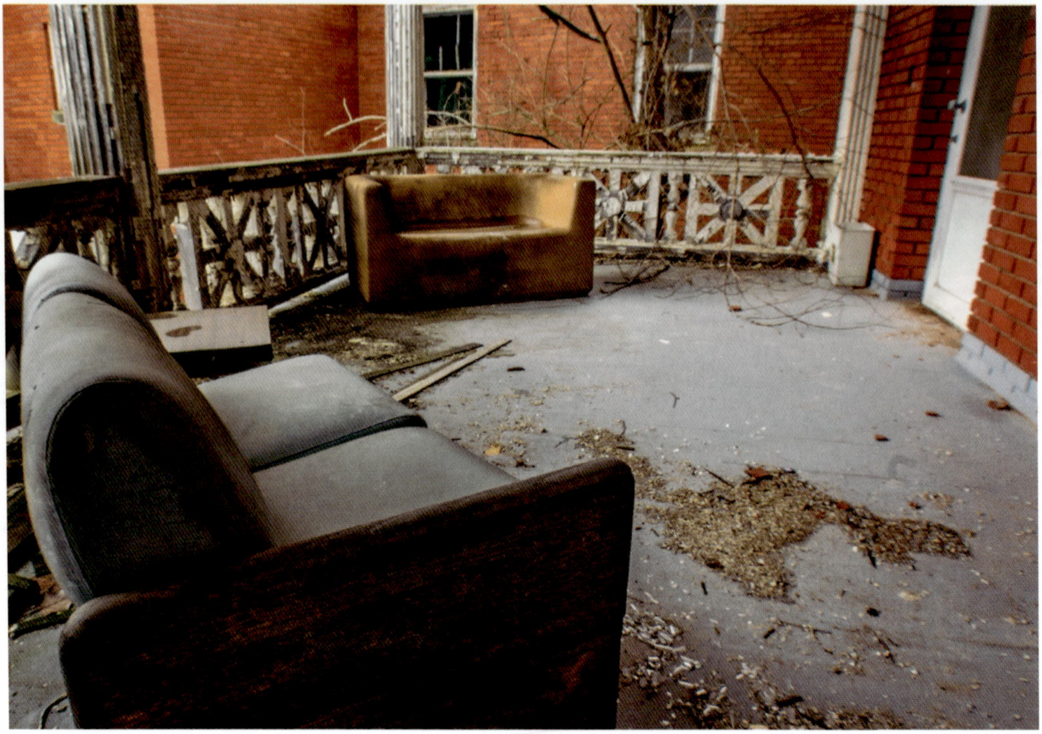

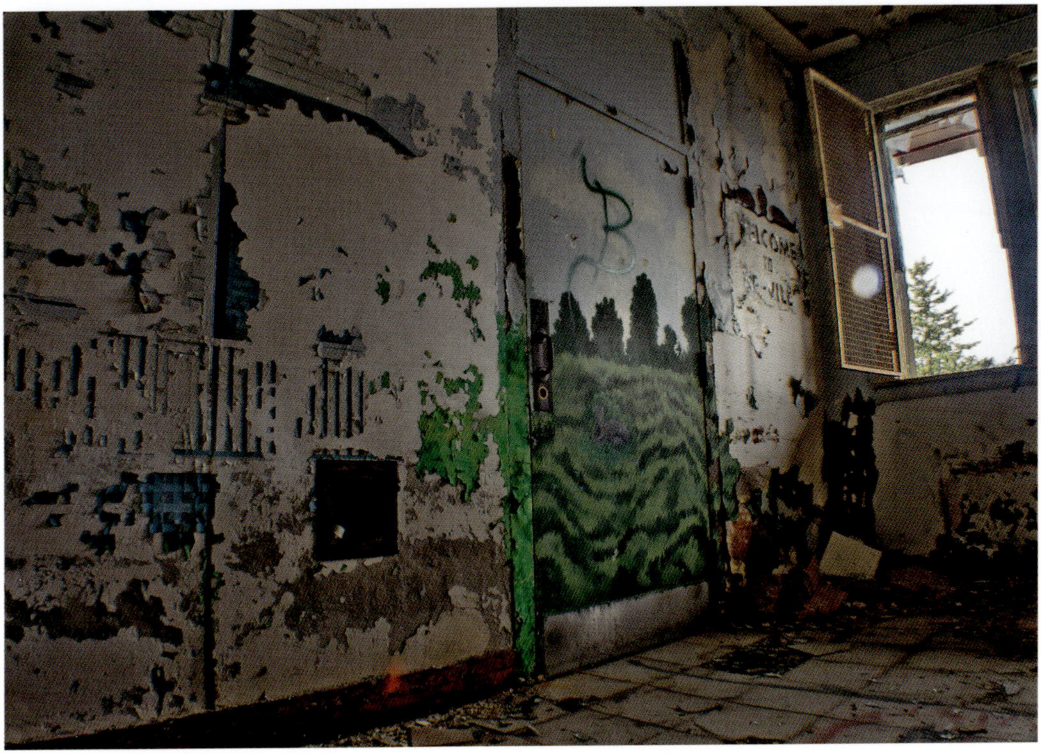

This is what is left of mural hall. A decrepit, peeling façade with barely recognizable lettering cries out the words, "WELCOME TO BE-VILLE." *[Photo by Brian Cray]*

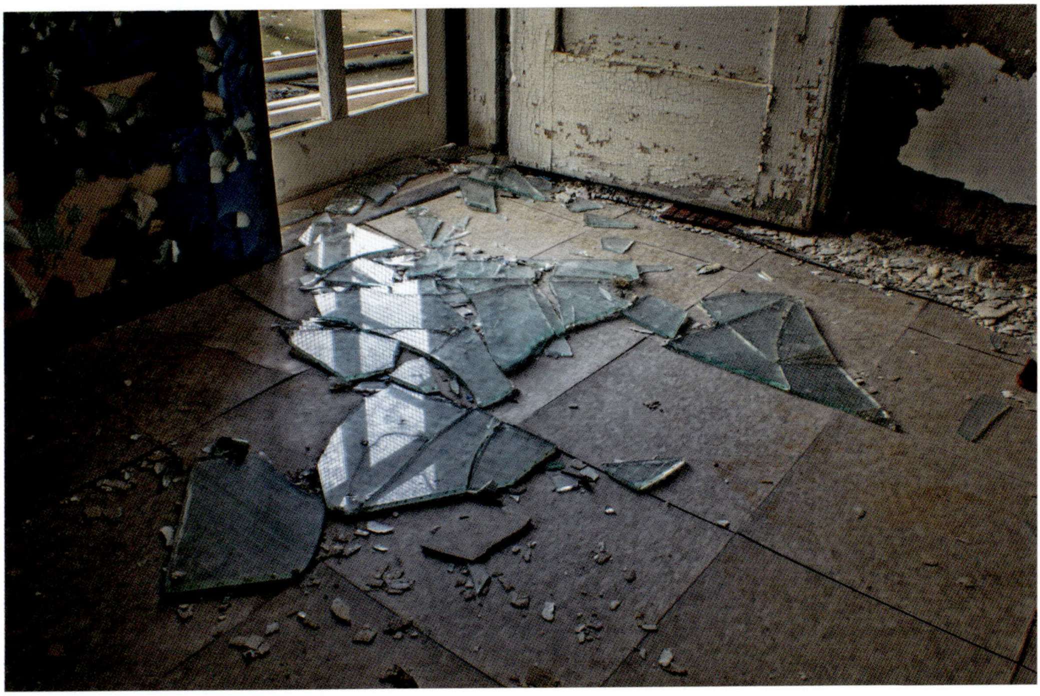

I can only see her broken reflection colored in shards of glass scattered along the floor. *[Photo by Brian Cray]*

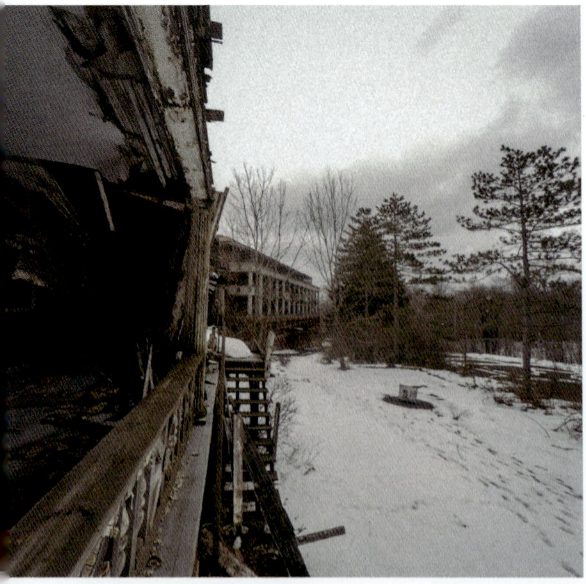

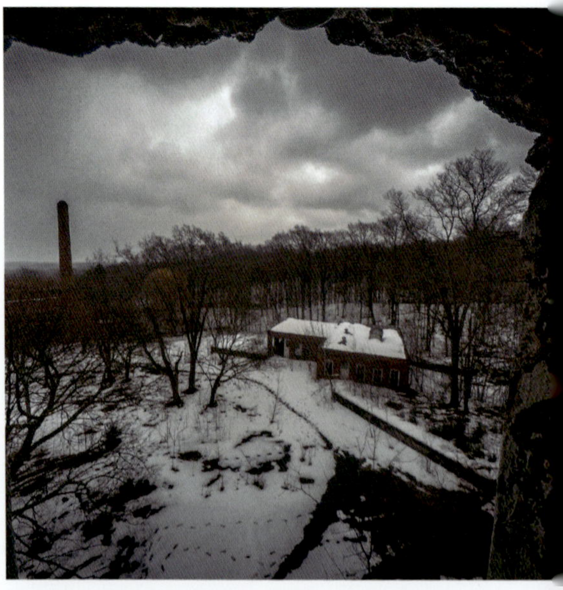

Above left: The grain only adds to the calamity of the walls and her ultimate decay. My explorations take me further into her past, and I save the best for last. *[Photo by Brian Cray]*

Above right: I gaze down at the Carpenter's Shop (Building #18) through the framing of loose bricks, and beneath the flat, monstrous sky. It's nothing like my last visit. *[Photo by Brian Cray]*

BUILDING #18 – CARPENTER'S SHOP

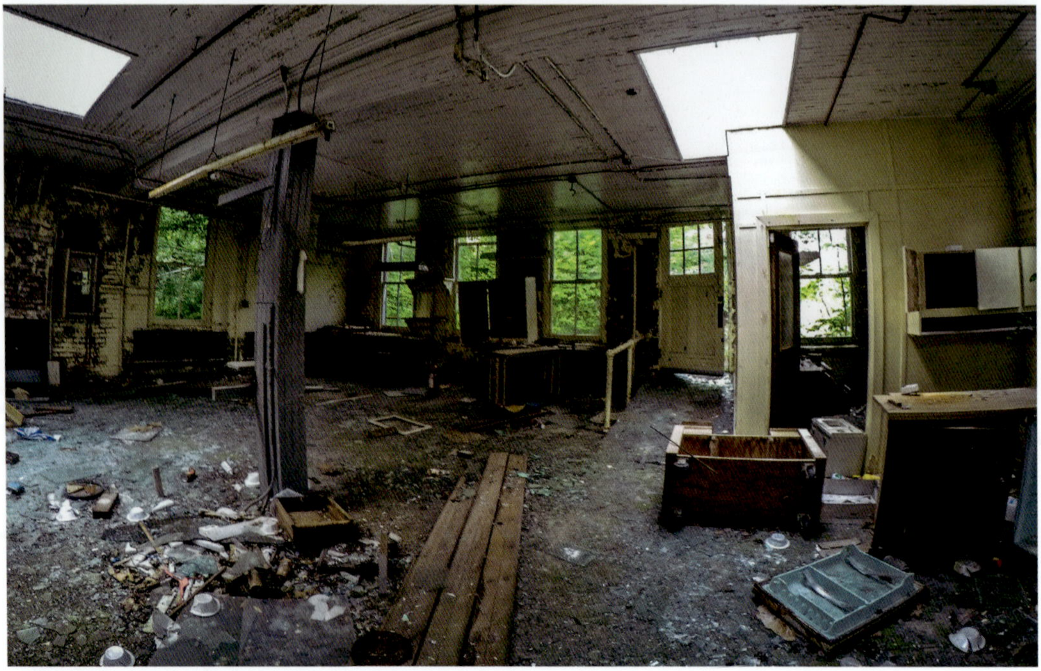

In 2016, the effervescent glow of springtime lit her dark cavities unmasking her wounds. You won't find a tool inside these empty walls. All that is left are loose boards, crumbs of glass and broken memories. *[Photo by Brian Cray]*

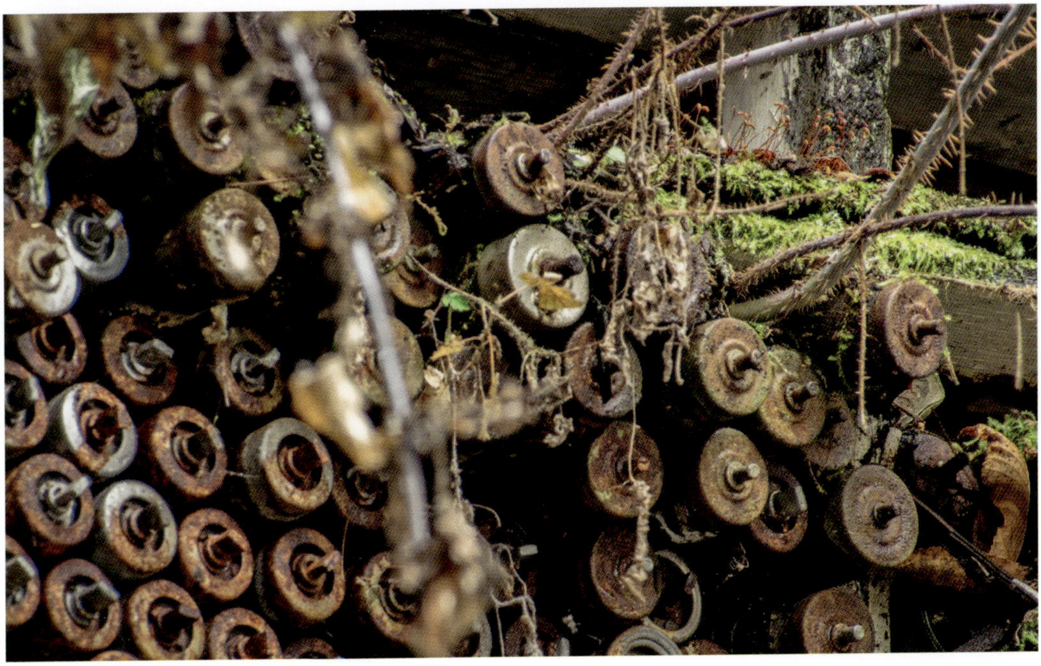

Fluorescent tubes rot in overgrown, prickly vines as moss breeds on the warped, wooden shelving. *[Photo by Brian Cray]*

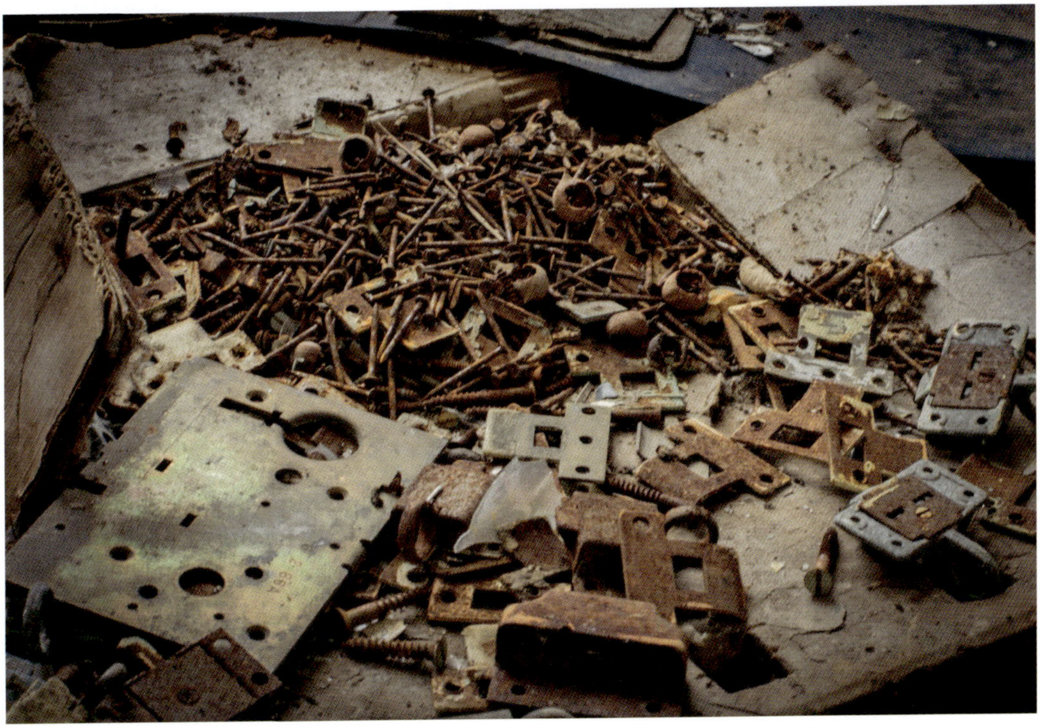

Piles of rusty nuts, bolts, nails, screws, sun-damaged cardboard and frail door hinges fester on a wooden work bench. I did not see a single tool in this building. I am sure vandals ransacked those goods long ago. *[Photo by Brian Cray]*

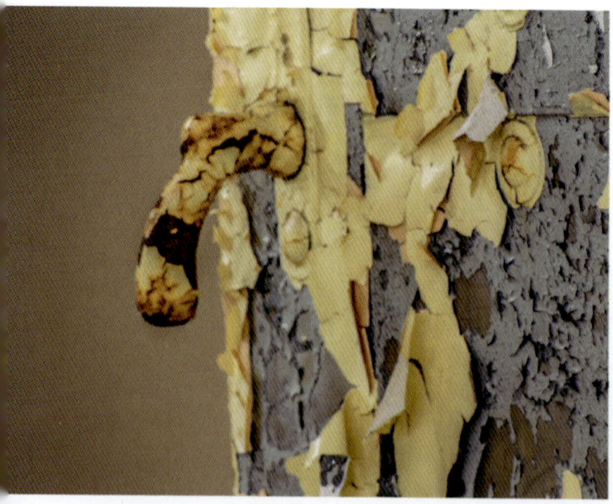

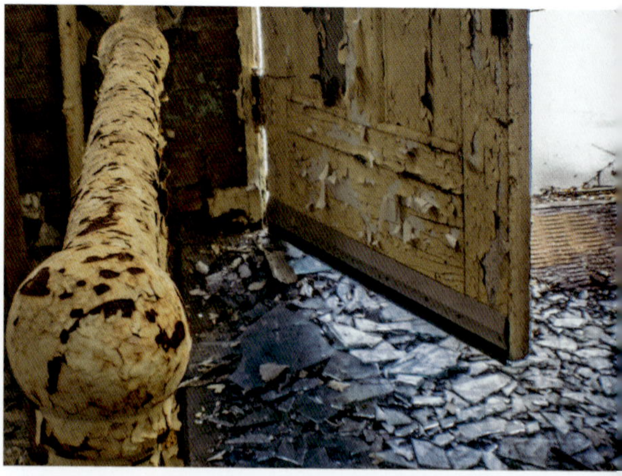

Above left: Moisture of the seasons peels back her lead paint exposing her base to the plague of oxidation. The door handles stay locked from the decadence of time. *[Photo by Brian Cray]*

Above right: Under the peeling of paint and the fading of bricks, I see more shattered glass, gleaning as blue as the ocean. I step over her dying reflection and wander onward to explore the last building before the next snowstorm hits. *[Photo by Brian Cray]*

BUILDING #20 – THE POWERHOUSE

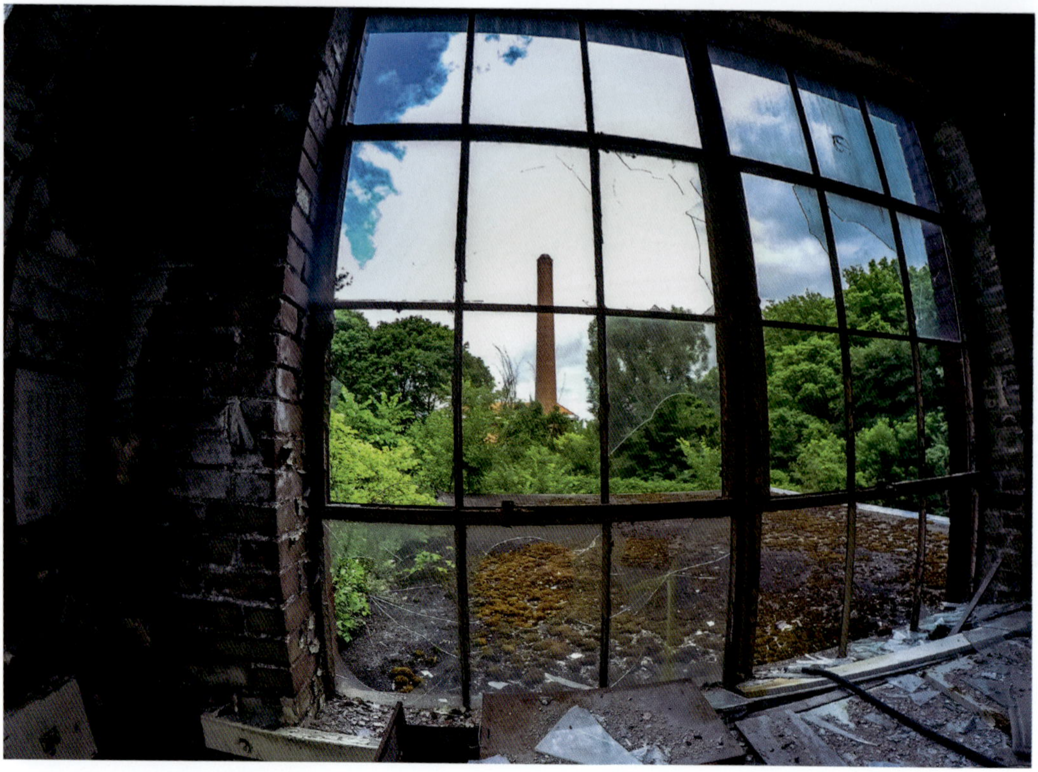

Through painted windows the creamy white clouds mask the baby blue sky and beyond the broken shards of glass, flakes of rust and asbestos, I feel the heart of the forest beating. Between the curving branches, I see smears of red brick and towering smokestack. *[Photo by Brian Cray]*

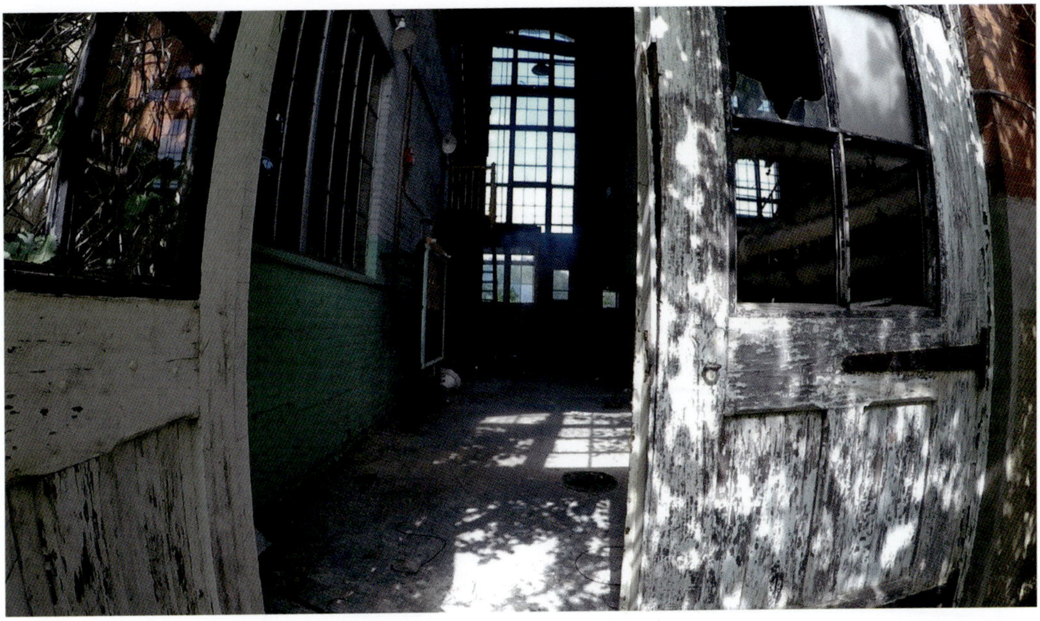

This is the POWERHOUSE! *[Photo by Brian Cray]*

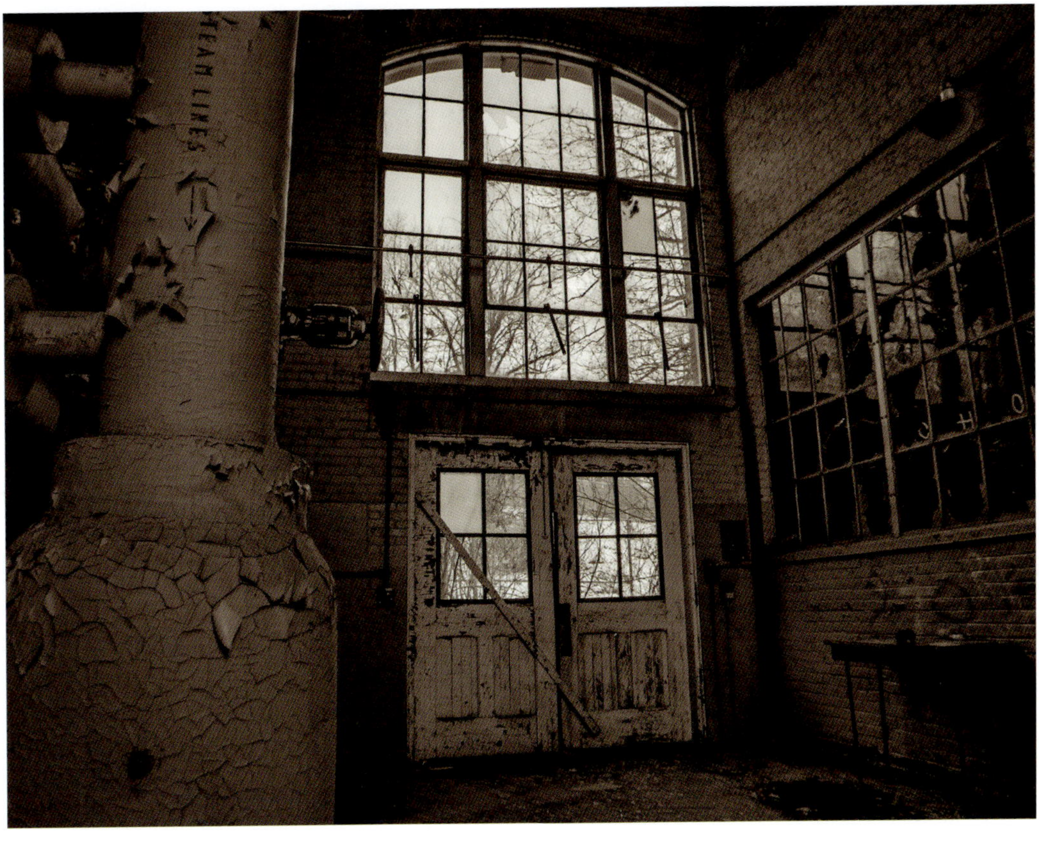

A sudden creak from the door startles me. I turn around, listening to the sweet silence of decay. I see the paint peeling back around me and focus on the arched windows feeding her light on this dismal day. *[Photo by Brian Cray]*

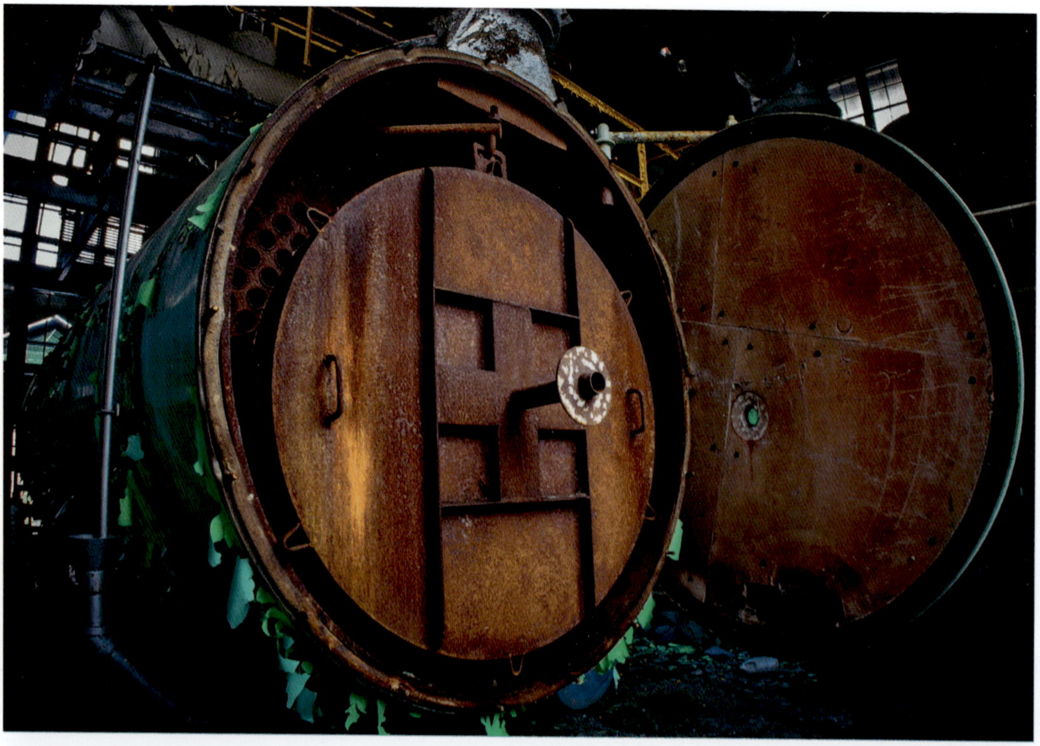

Streaks of orange and brown oxidation speckle the insides of the boiler. I reach out and clasp my hand among the gritty rung, but her sharp teeth tickle my palms as if goading me to step back. *[Photo by Brian Cray]*

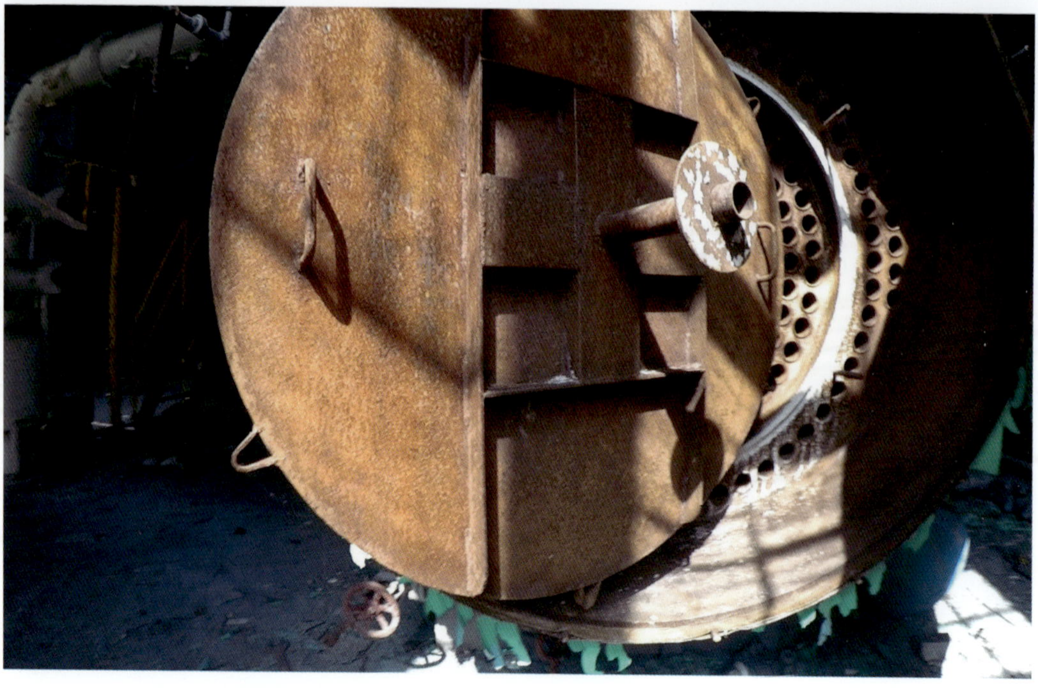

A heavy iron disk dangles in the air spiking my curiosity to peek inside. But inside the dark cylindrical walls, I only see tinier, ominous cavities. *[Photo by Brian Cray]*

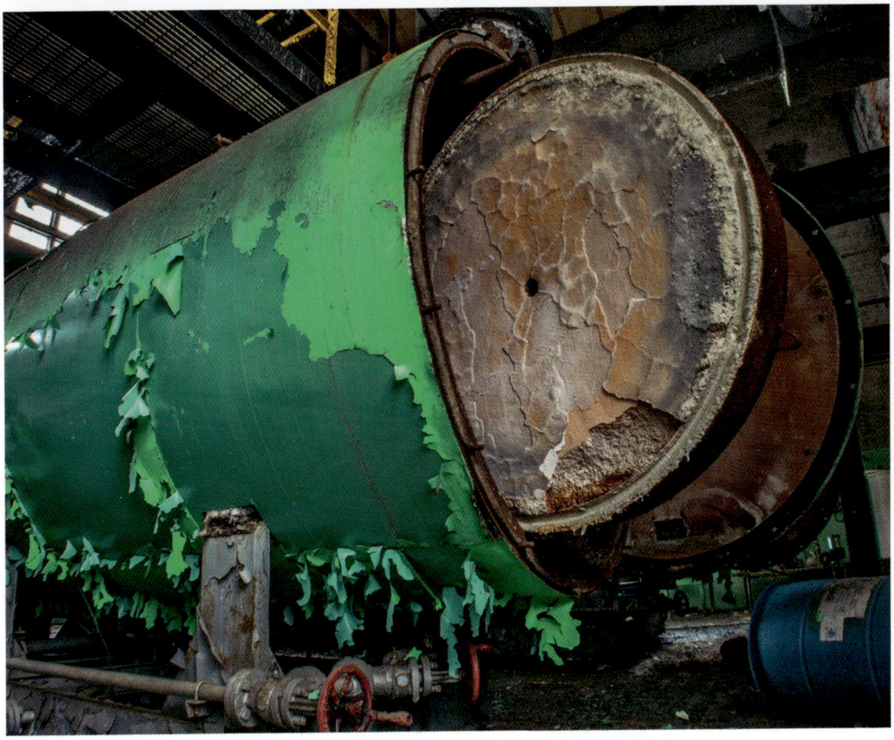

Above: One Ames Steam Boiler is big enough to carry the total load of the coldest winter day. Natural gas was readily available as the municipal hospital was located on a national storage field where eight gas wells resided ("Perrysburg Campus Property," 1989). *[Photo by Brian Cray]*

Below left: Teel paint buds off the line of boilers with her metal slowly drooping to the floor as my eyes reach the far wall of the powerhouse. *[Photo by Brian Cray]*

Below right: The blurs and streaks complement the whirs and creaks in a downtrodden beauty of hopelessness. *[Photo by Brian Cray]*

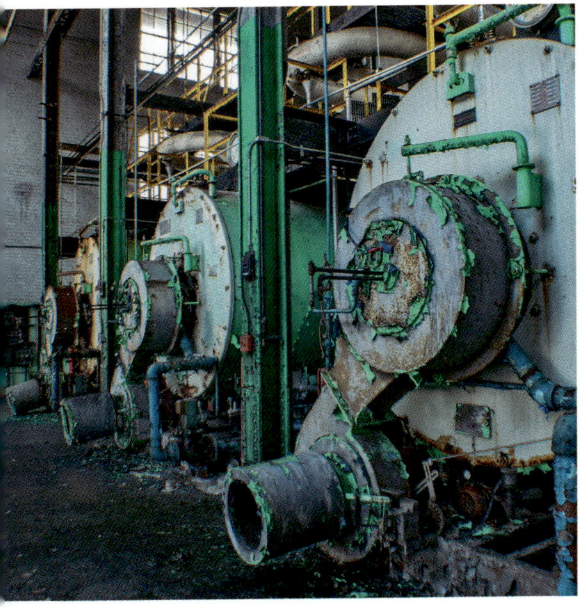

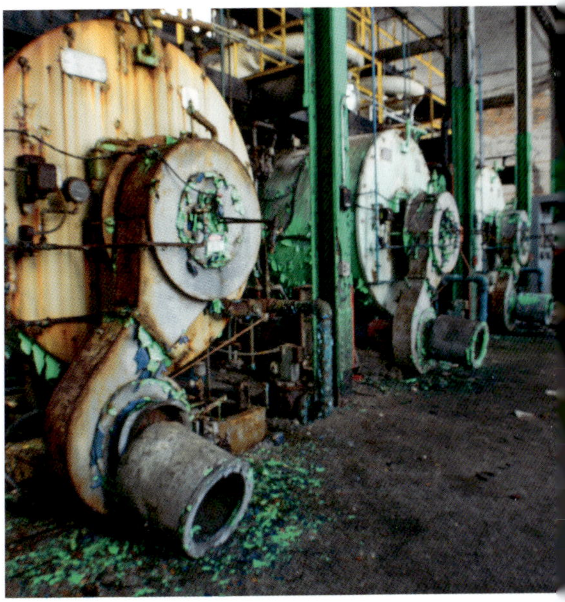

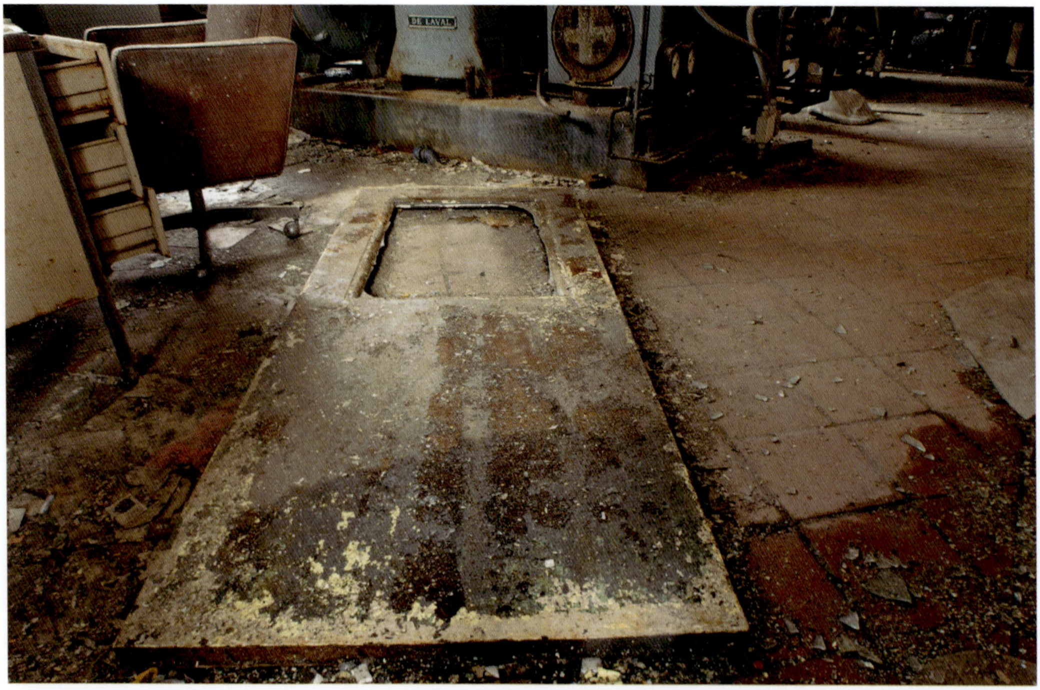

The door lays there infected by bitter decay as pools of grease and films of dust gut the grains of splintered wood. *[Photo by Brian Cray]*

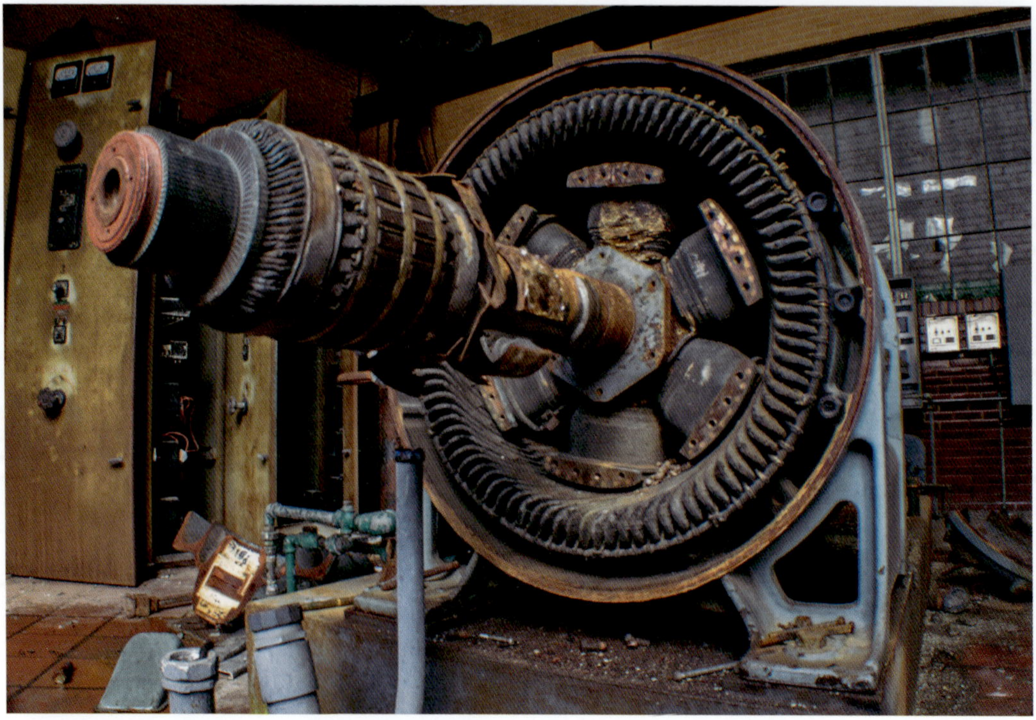

The gears of life dwindle with time and there is no conjuring to conserve one's strapping youth. Her time is near. *[Photo by Brian Cray]*

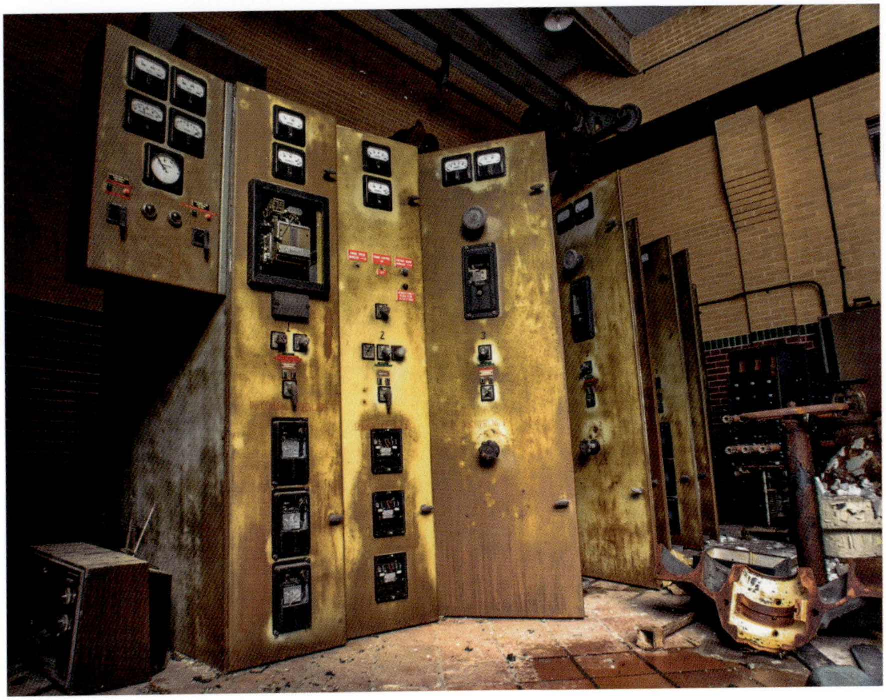

Stained yellow doors distract my eyes from the lifeless gauges on the backup electric generator used only for emergency power, which was installed in 1960 ("Perrysburg Campus Property," 1989). *[Photo by Brian Cray]*

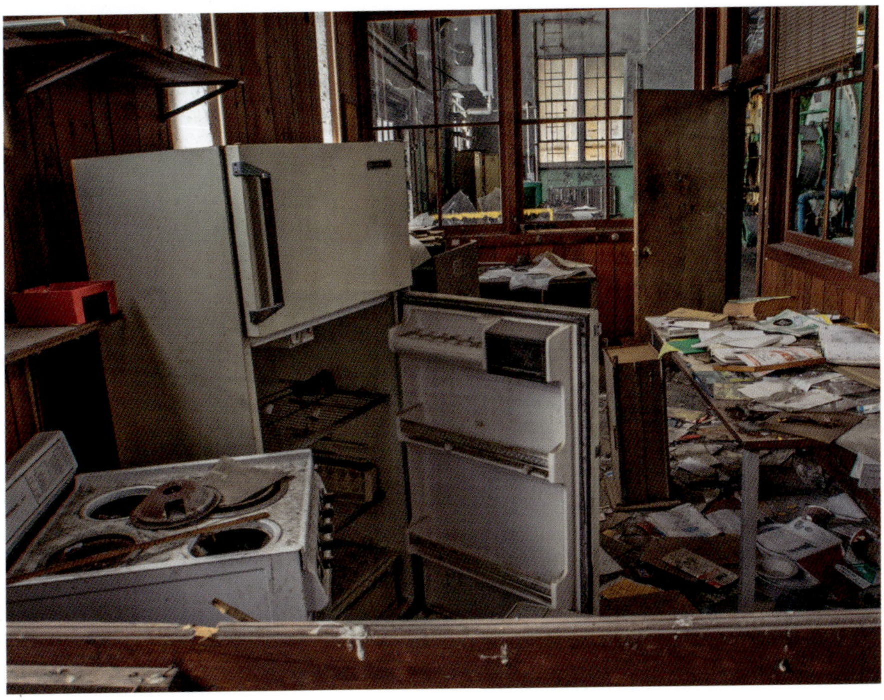

Open pages left astray plague the floor and desks of the employee powerhouse lounge. If you want to use the fridge or stove, you'll have to think again—it looks like a bear ransacked the place. *[Photo by Brian Cray]*

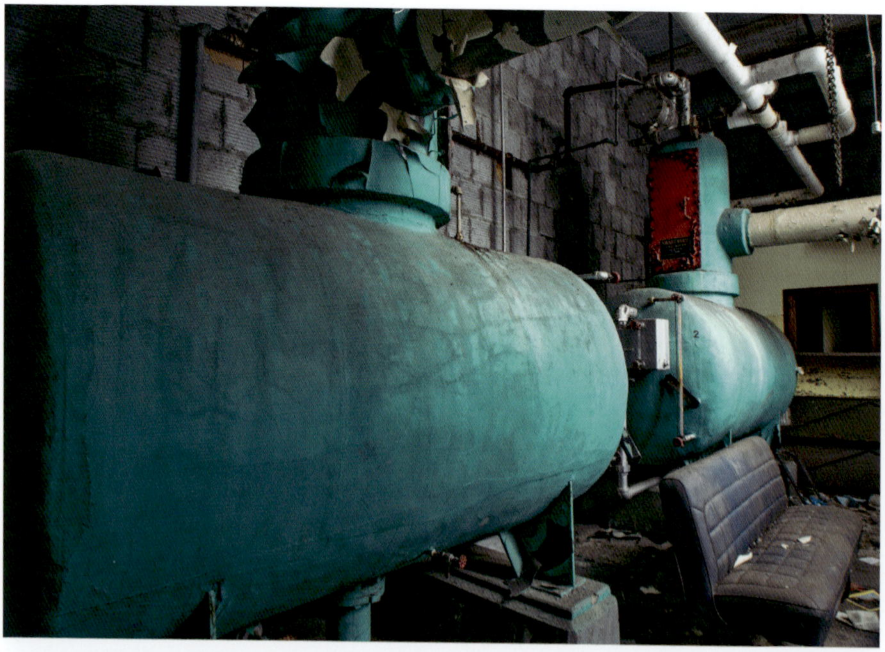

Beyond the chips of faded blue paint it all boils down to proverbial age. Each of these hot water tanks held 1,000 gallons of water, which were heated by exhaust steam, providing hot water for the upwards of 400 patients and full laundry ("Perrysburg Campus Property," 1989). *[Photo by Brian Cray]*

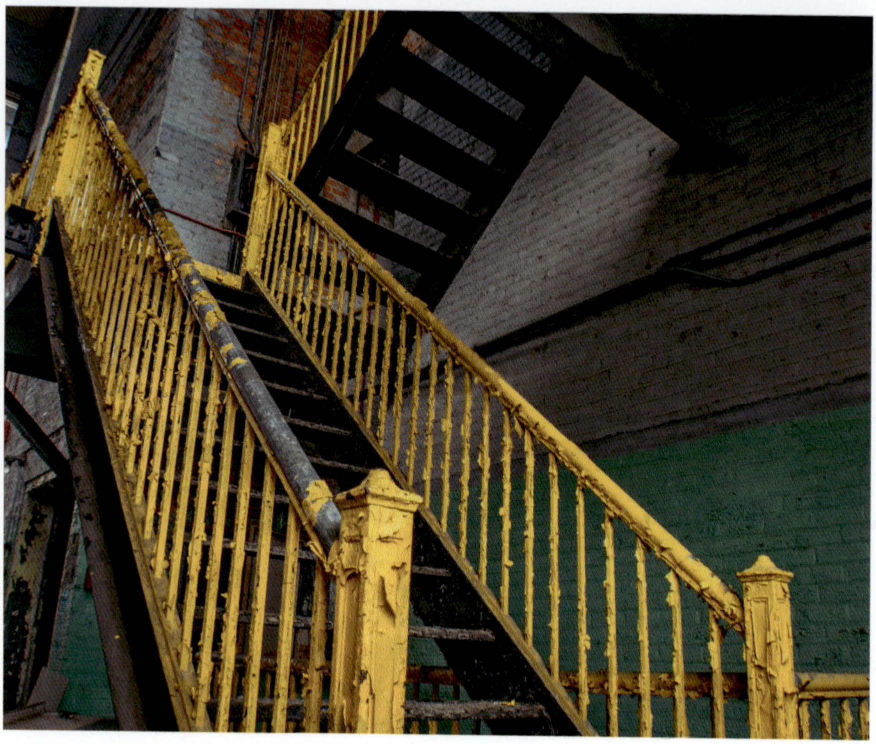

I wanted to find the Land of Oz. So I followed the yellow stairwell to the top, only to stop at the face of a lock, gripping the horseshoe rung of metal, held me from the roof altogether. *[Photo by Brian Cray]*

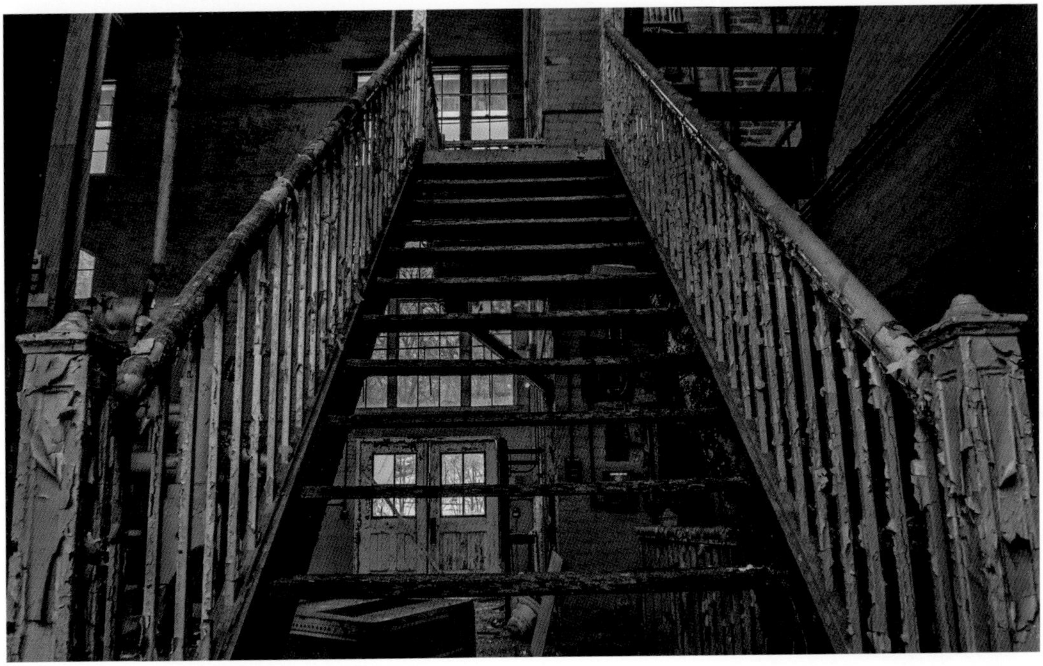

Between the metal treads are open spaces. Through the decay, I stand still just smelling the musty dampness of the room. My eyes venture to the top of the stairwell and I can only wonder how often workers tramped to the top to smoke on the roof. *[Photo by Brian Cray]*

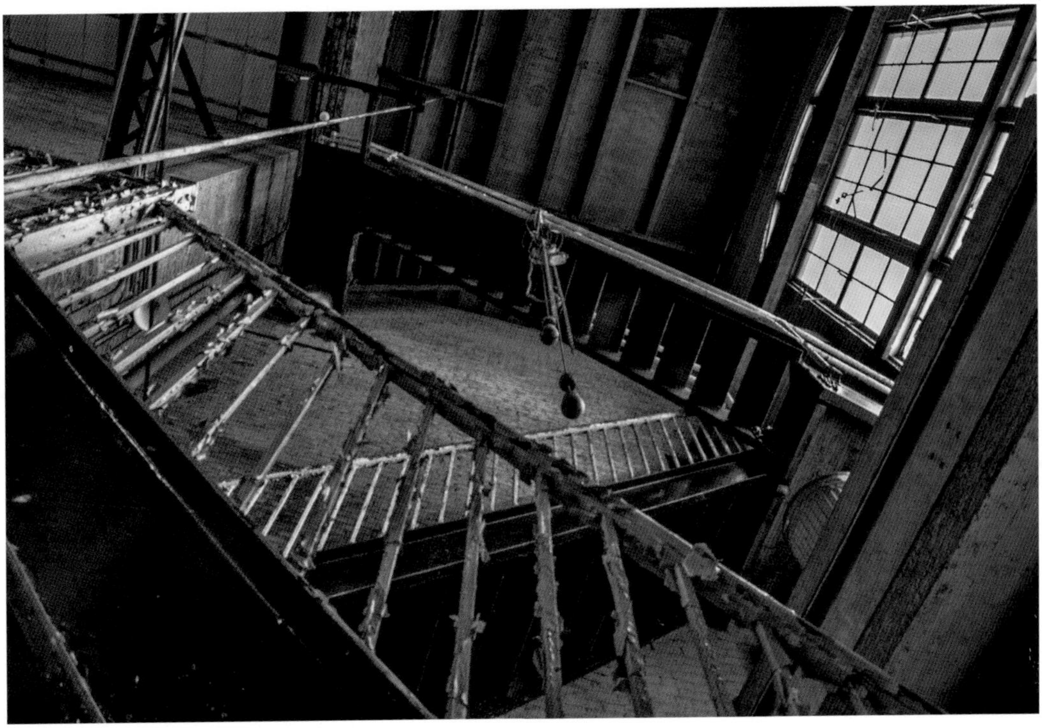

The balls and chains distract me from the zigzagging balustrade leading to the top of this behemoth. *[Photo by Brian Cray]*

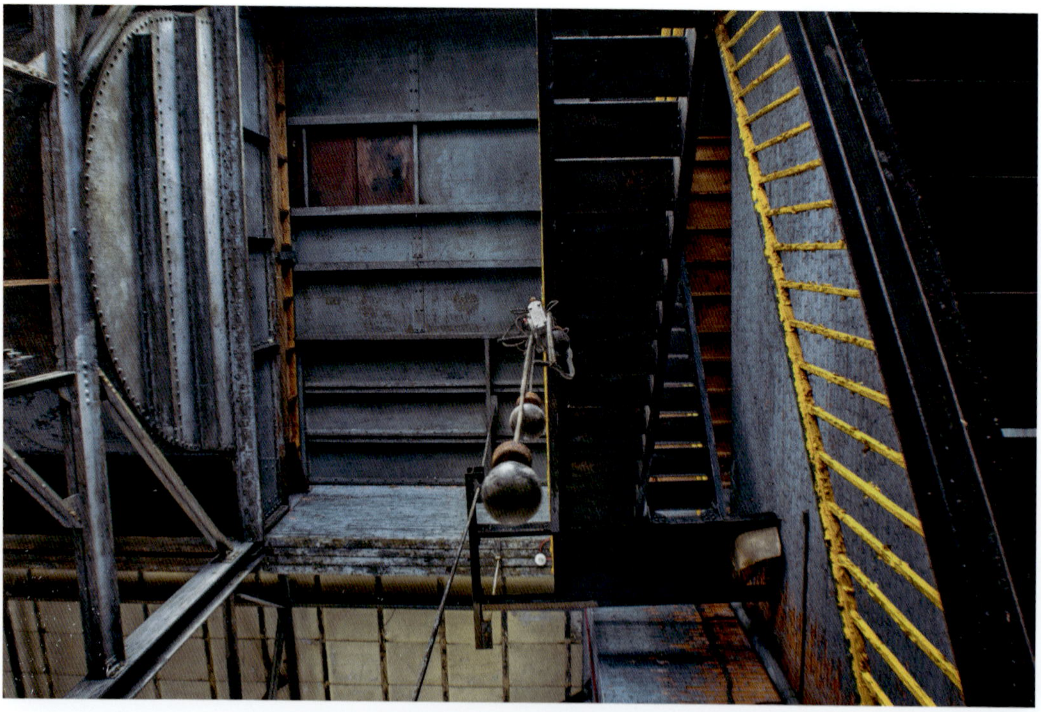

Her ceiling stares down at me in despair as her walls shed the illusion of life. It's nothing more than slow decay as nature peels back layers of stone paint and waits. *[Photo by Brian Cray]*

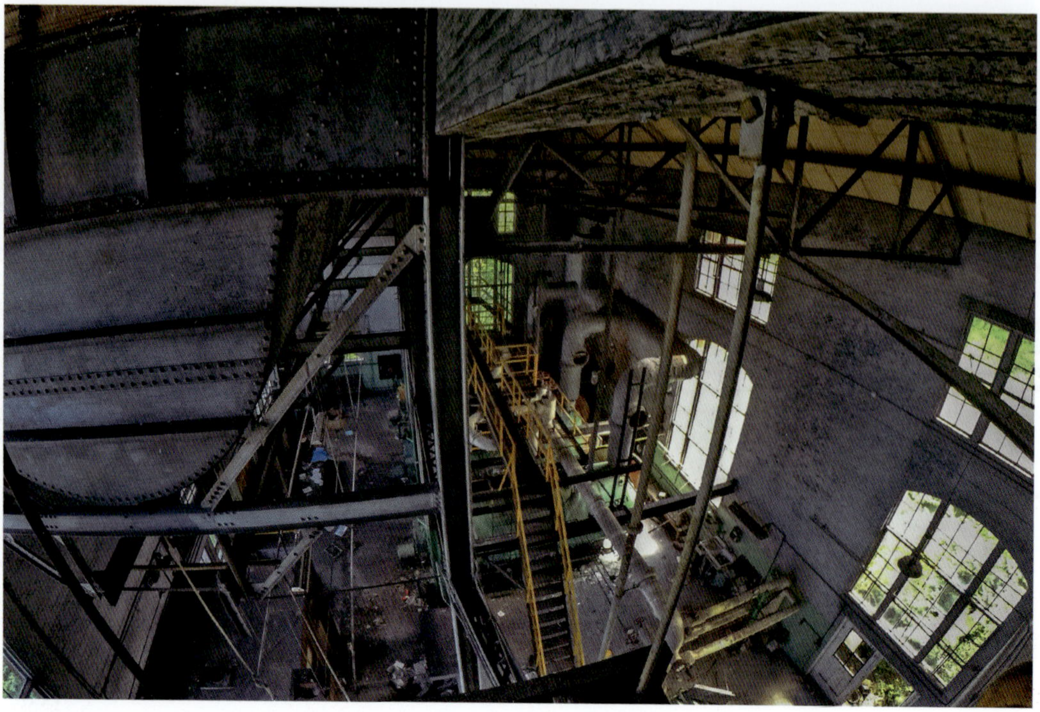

From the fourth flight of stairs I peer out across the powerhouse. I close my eyes and I hear the steam system hissing, the boilers chugging like freight trains, and my imagination fills in the gaps of the past. *[Photo by Brian Cray]*

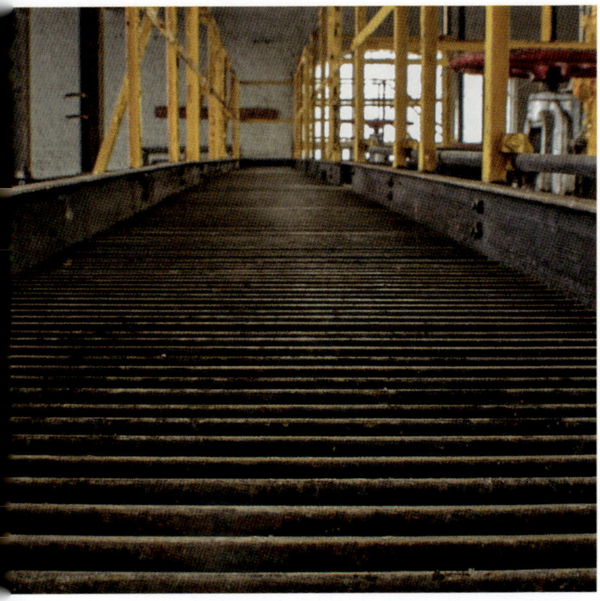

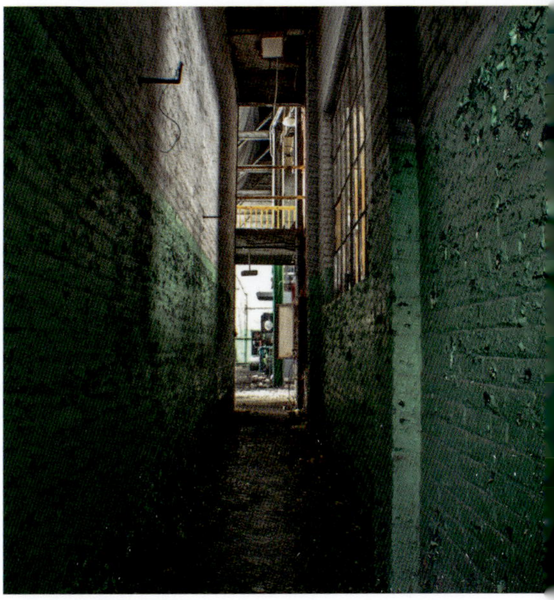

Above left: Beneath these metal treads the massive boilers lay to rest. *[Photo by Brian Cray]*

Above right: I wander the narrow corridor, between the peeling teal bricks, covering my nose from the pungent smell of asbestos. *[Photo by Brian Cray]*

Below: **"DANGER HAZARDOUS VOLTAGE INSIDE!"** Don't worry the power died out here long ago, but I didn't open any doors to find out either. *[Photo by Brian Cray]*

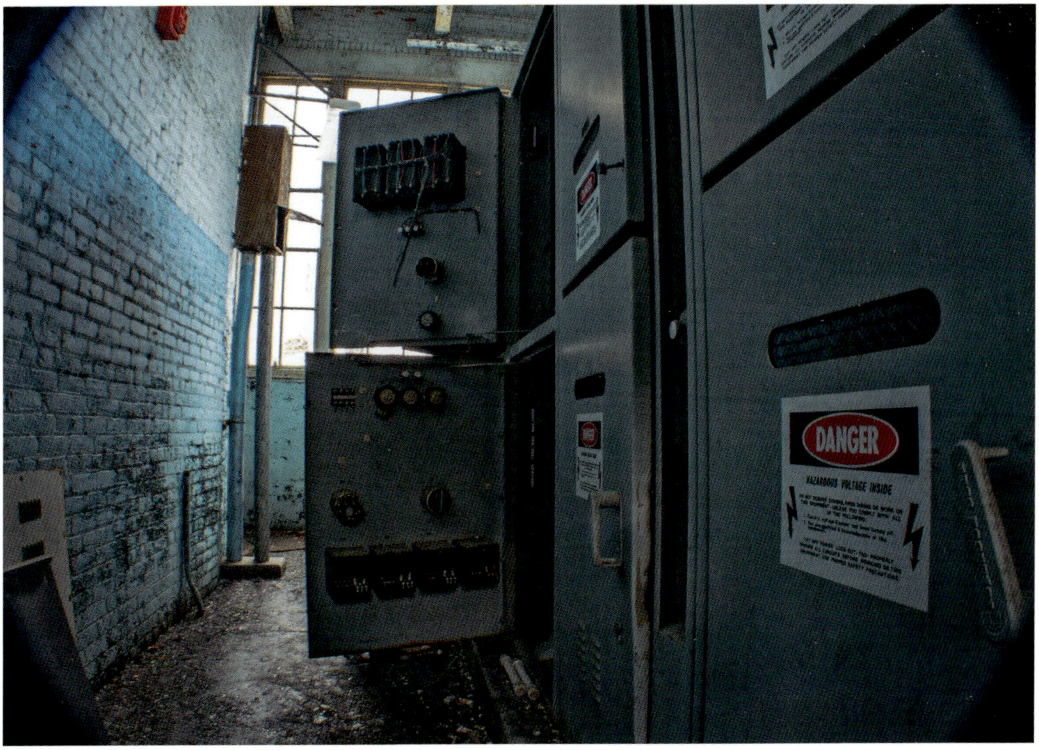

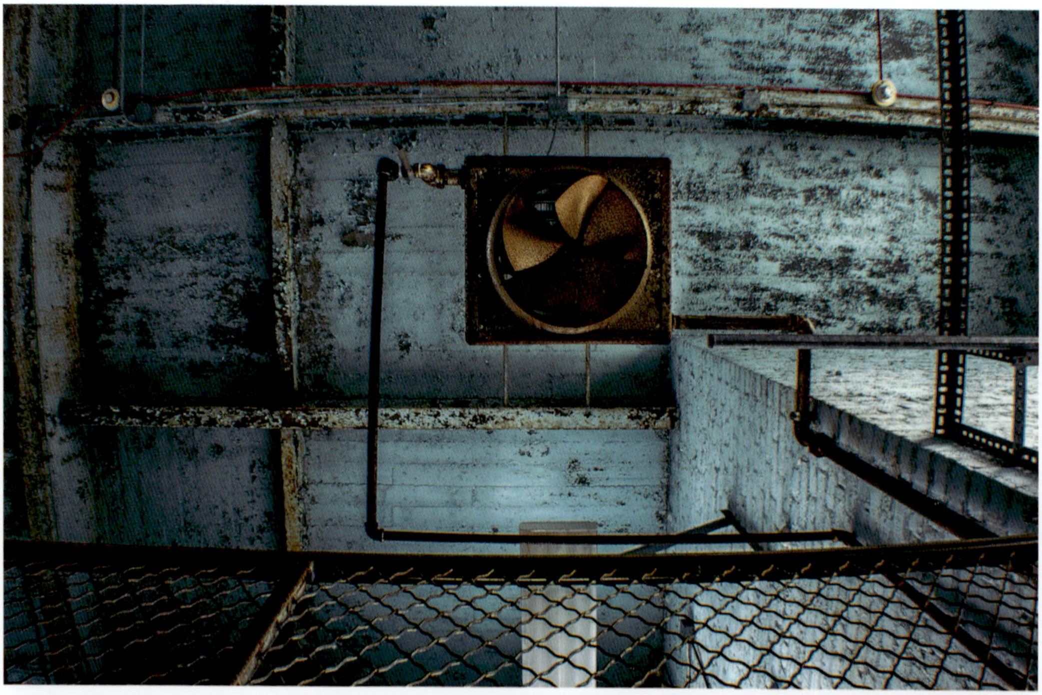

As I look up at the rusted blades, I feel the canvas of winter touch my soul. Blue chills cry down from the ceiling and suddenly it begins to snow outside. *[Photo by Brian Cray]*

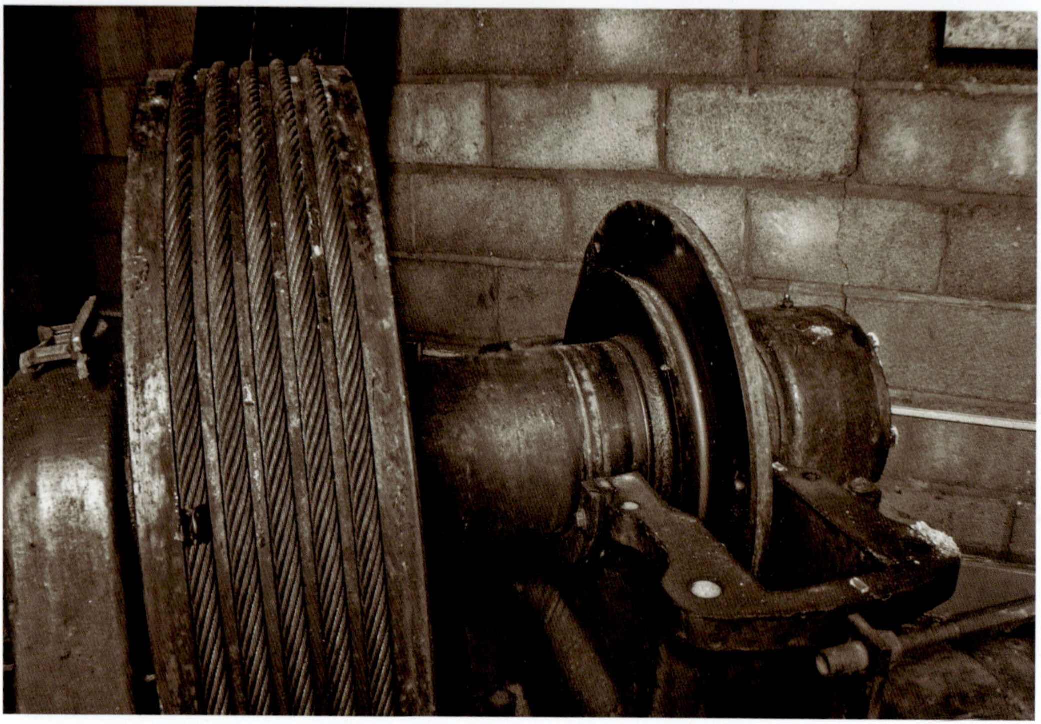

My eyes traverse the grooves of thick cable mesmerized by steel and the sheer size of this gear. *[Photo by Brian Cray]*

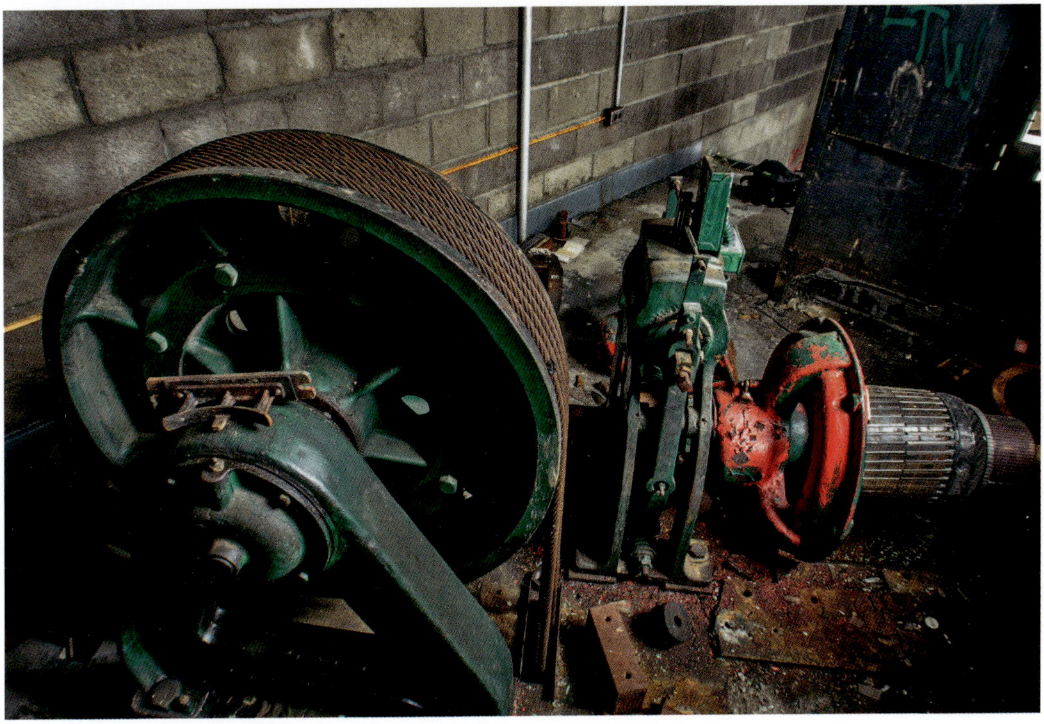

My feet feel the safest by this gear, safer than any floor, except the ground floor. *[Photo by Brian Cray]*

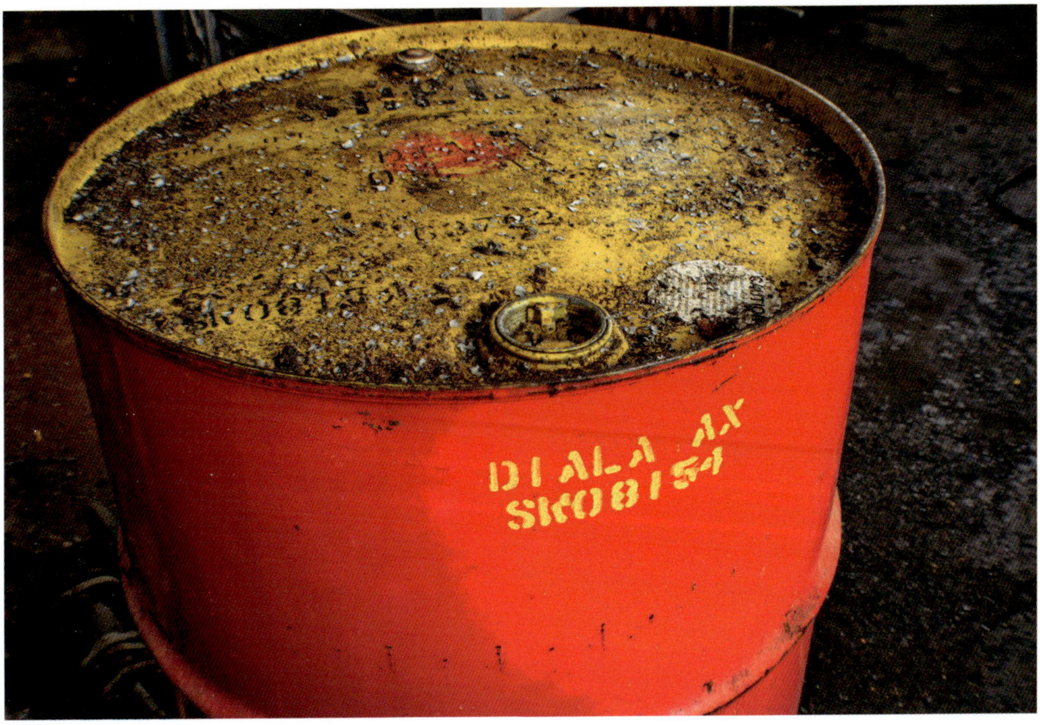

As I continue to piddle through vacant rooms, I stumble upon a steel drum with the letters "DI ALA AX SK08154," an old oil drum. *[Photo by Brian Cray]*

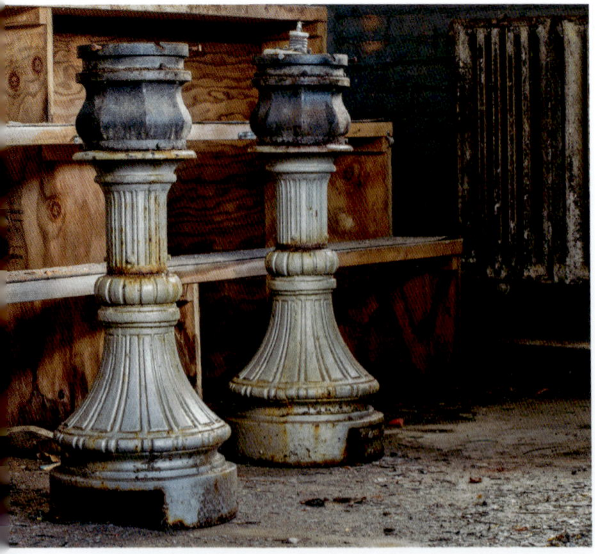

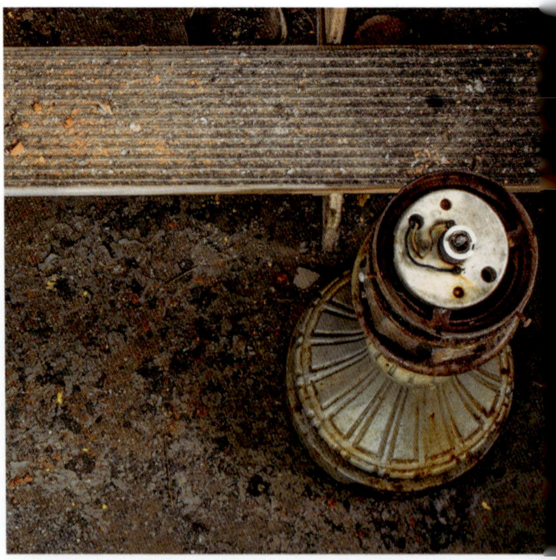

Above left: Beyond the oil drum I locked my focus on these two stunning, silver, lamppost bases, slightly oxidized from age. *[Photo by Brian Cray]*

Above right: Paint chips and flakes of brick speckle the floor like autumn leaves as my eyes explore the depths of the light fixtures below. *[Photo by Brian Cray]*

BUILDING #6

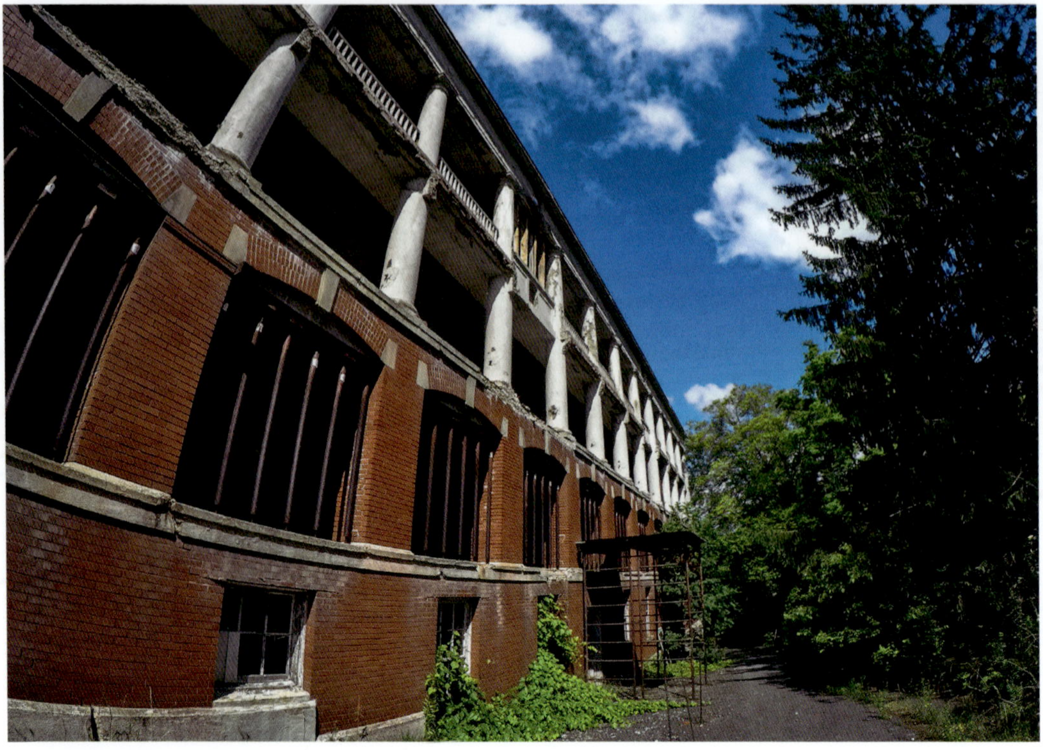

Building #6 was designed by Howard Beck and completed construction in 1924. *[Photo by Brian Cray]*

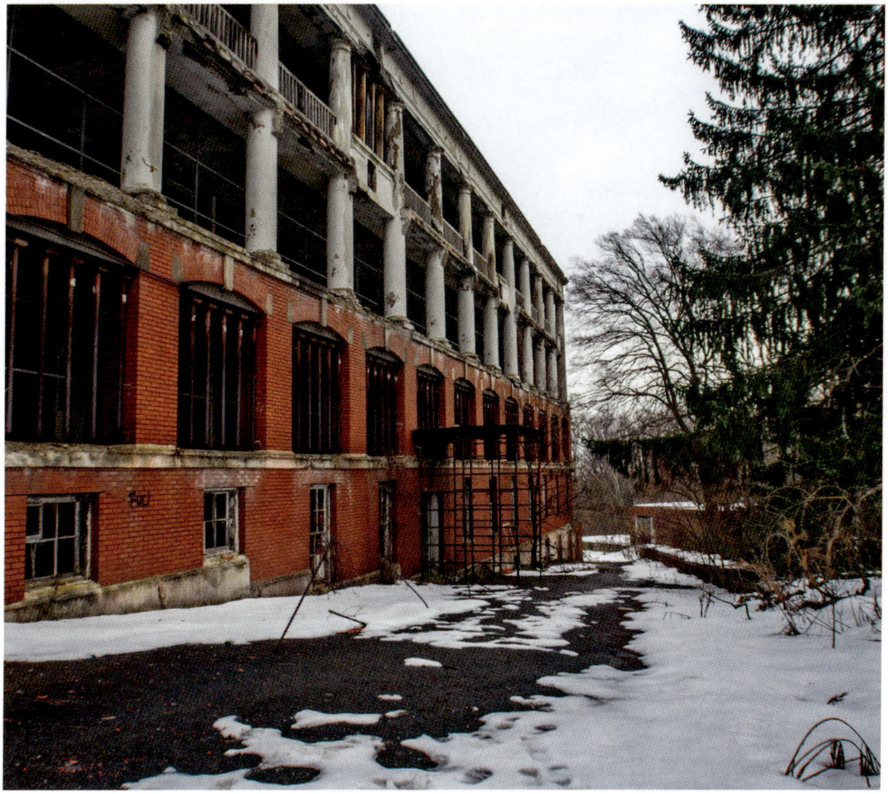

I stand in the same spot just two years after previous visit during the brutal month of December, looking out at Building #6 in the eye of winter. *[Photo by Brian Cray]*

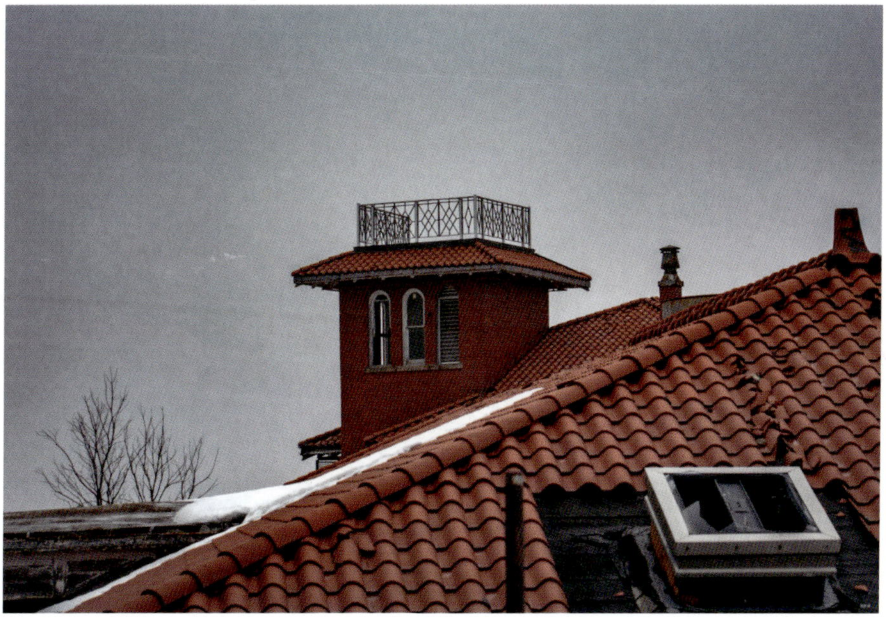

Shortly, I would find my way up to the distant patio after wandering her many vacant rooms. *[Photo by Brian Cray]*

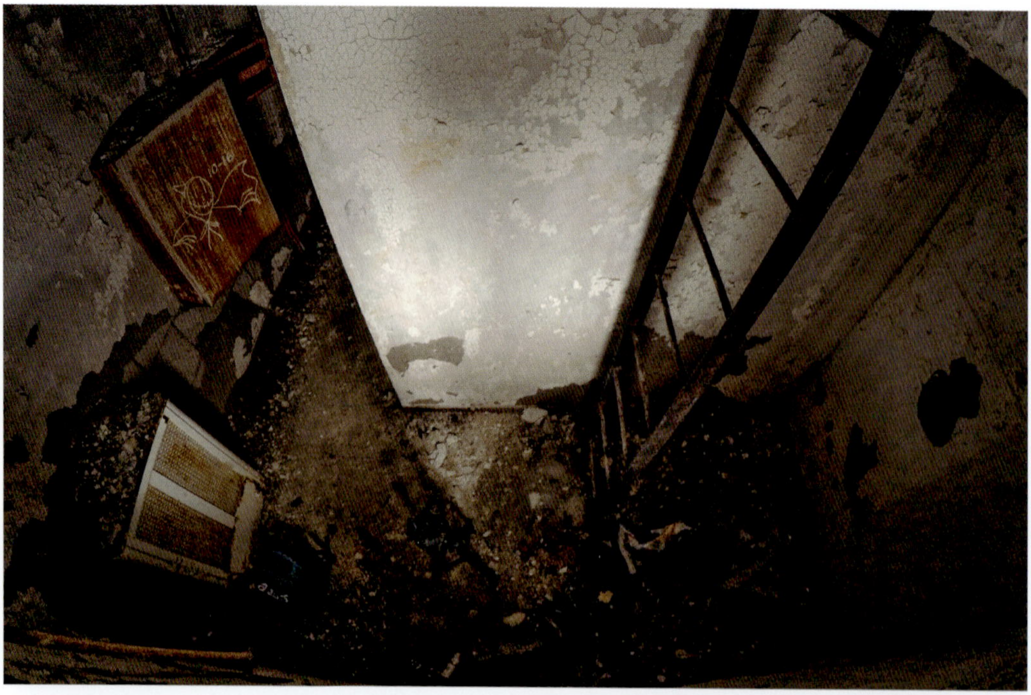

I don't believe in apparitions or paranormal activity, but the noises, the creaking doors and screaming windows, choked my intuitions. "Just follow the ladder," I thought. *[Photo by Brian Cray]*

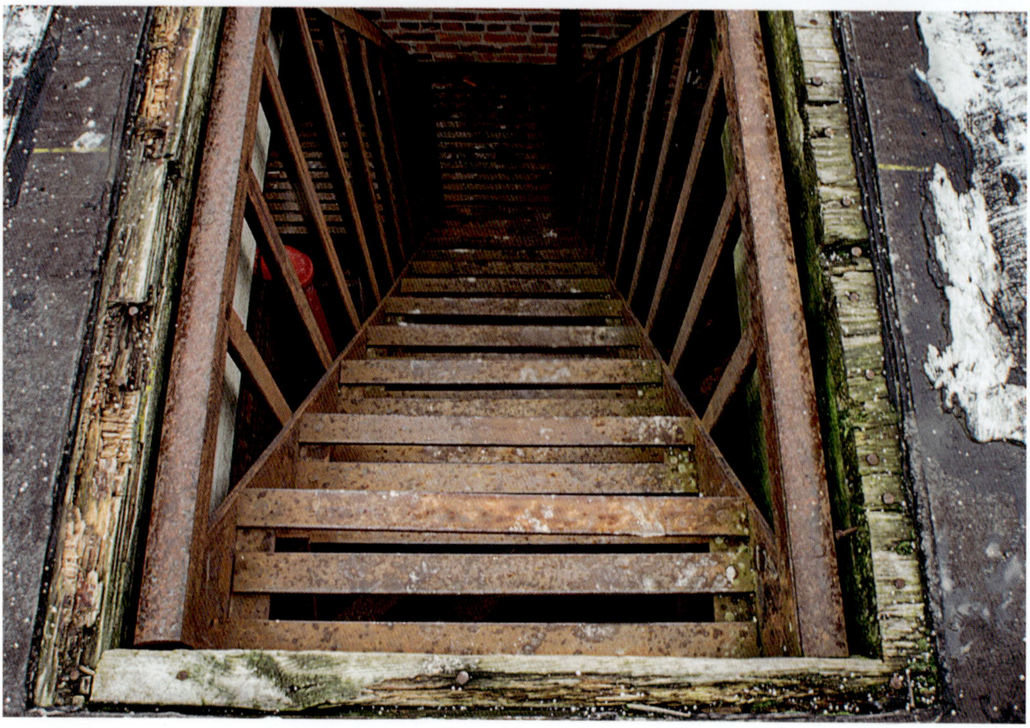

I meander up the rusty steps. My feet creak with each slow plunge upward as I wander the endless maze of stairs to her rooftop. *[Photo by Brian Cray]*

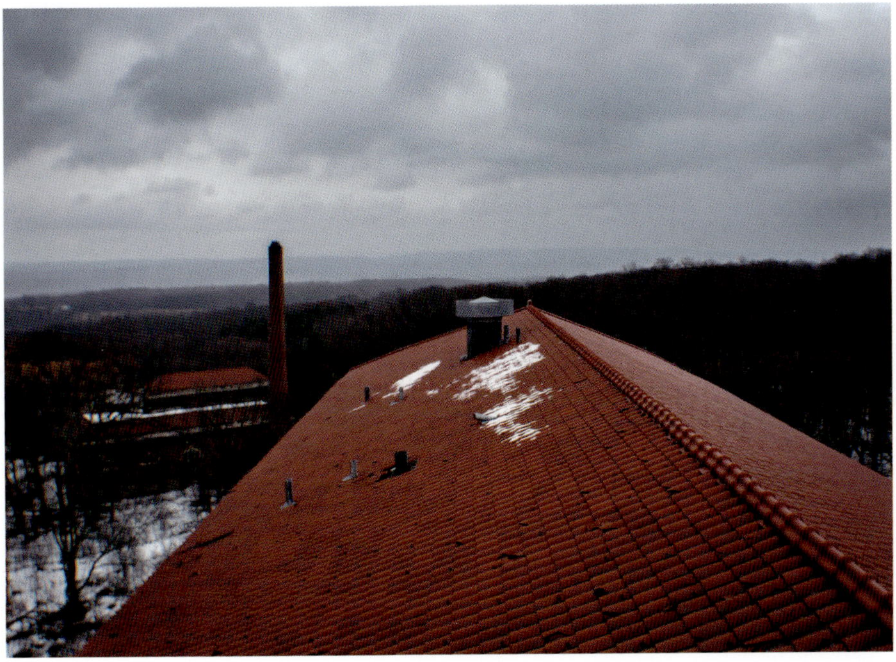

The hipped spine of clay tiles shoots off towards the Allegheny Mountains. Somewhere behind the clouds, beyond the lifeless trees, rests one of the frozen Great Lakes and the Canadian shoreline. *[Photo by Brian Cray]*

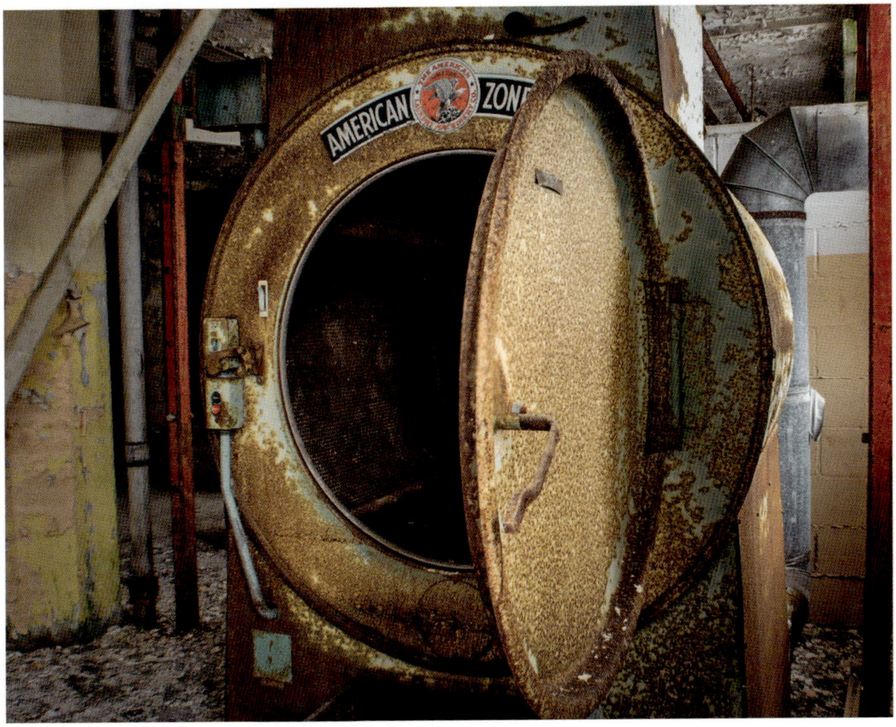

Lesions spread across the coarse metal like the White Plague. I can only wonder what the rest of this ward holds within her fading walls. *[Photo by Brian Cray]*

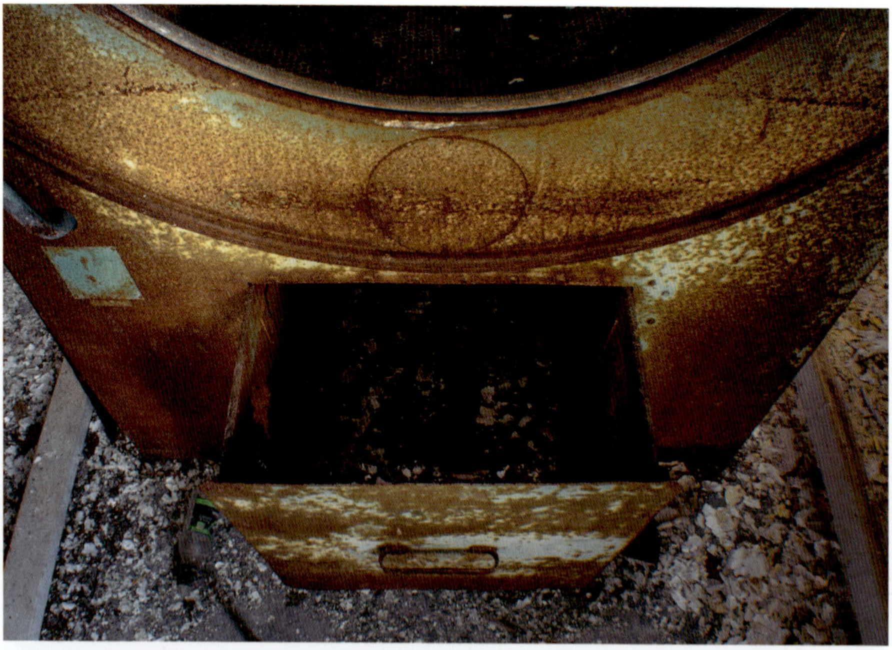

I look down at the drawer to the industrial dryer, completely rusted shut, and festering with asbestos. It only gets worse as I wander further onward. *[Photo by Brian Cray]*

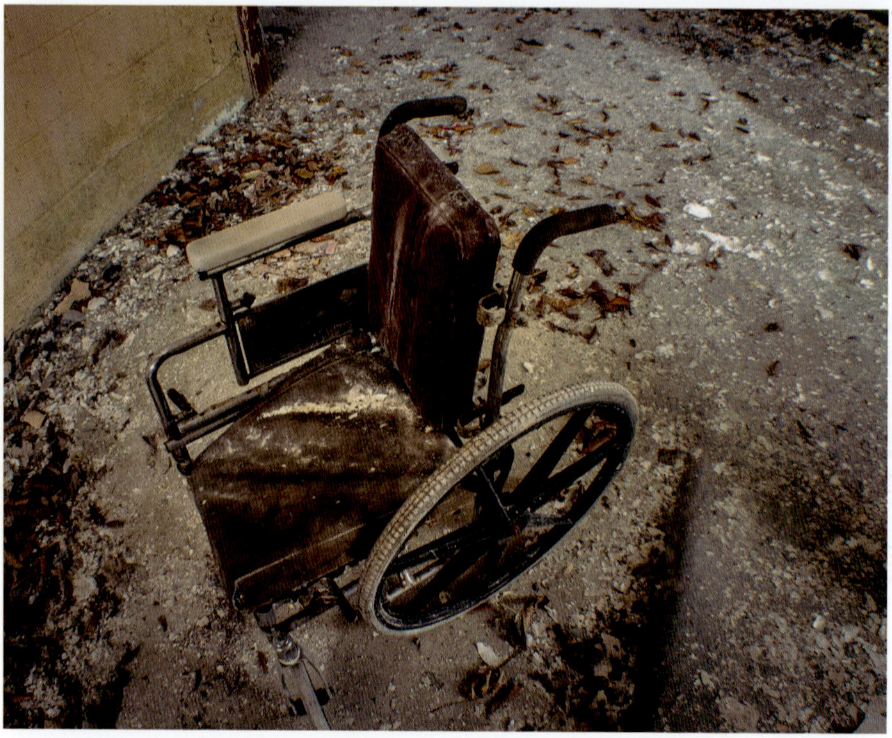

I shut my eyes and imagine the blur of suffering faces who once sat in this very wheelchair. I imagine the morose thoughts that infected their minds much like the contagion that plagued them. *[Photo by Brian Cray]*

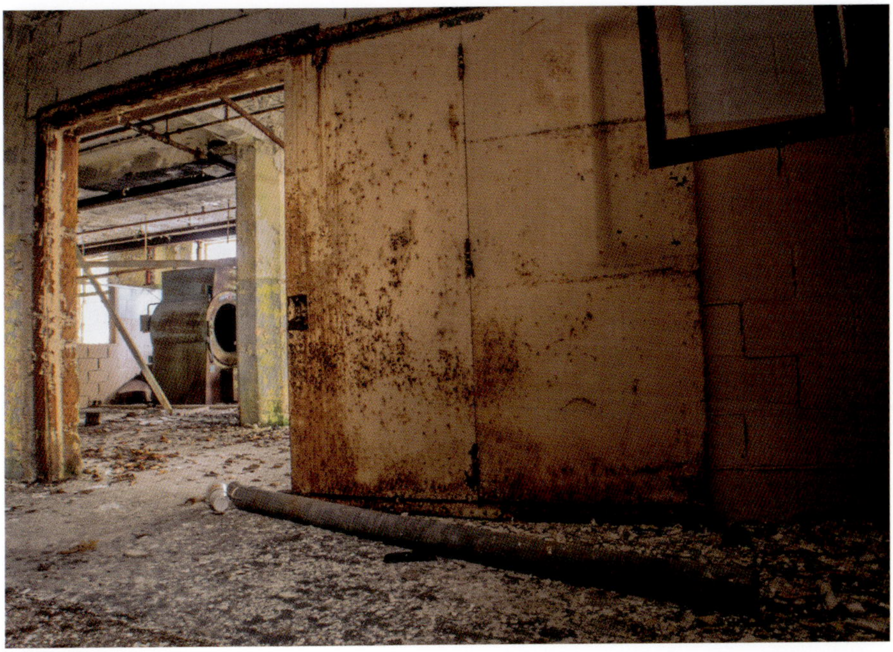

I turn around freeing my mind from her troubled past as I venture forward for the journey ahead of me. *[Photo by Brian Cray]*

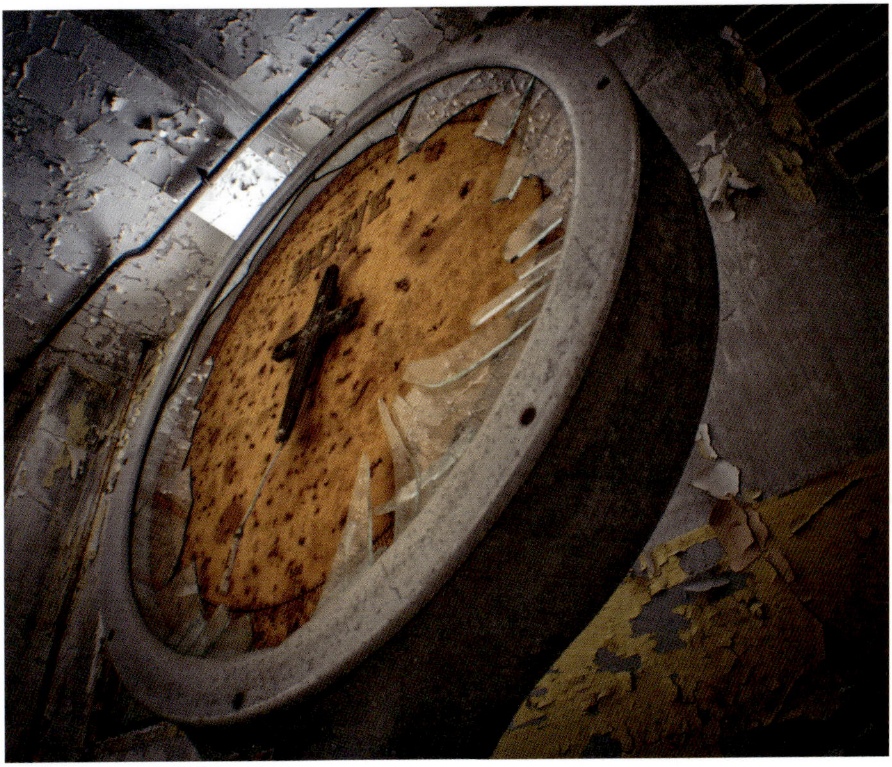

Sharp fingers orbit a scale that once weighed patients, but now she is only weighed down by the sonorous wrath of nature. *[Photo by Brian Cray]*

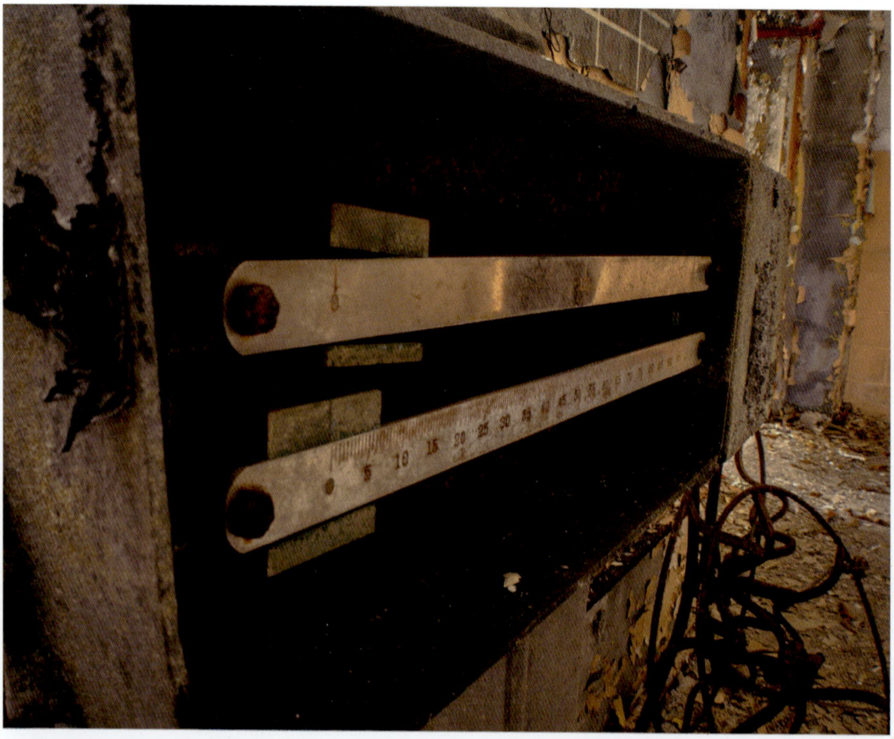

0 … 5 … 10 … 15 … 20 … 25 … 30 … the grainy numbers fade away joining the ruins of a lost cause. *[Photo by Brian Cray]*

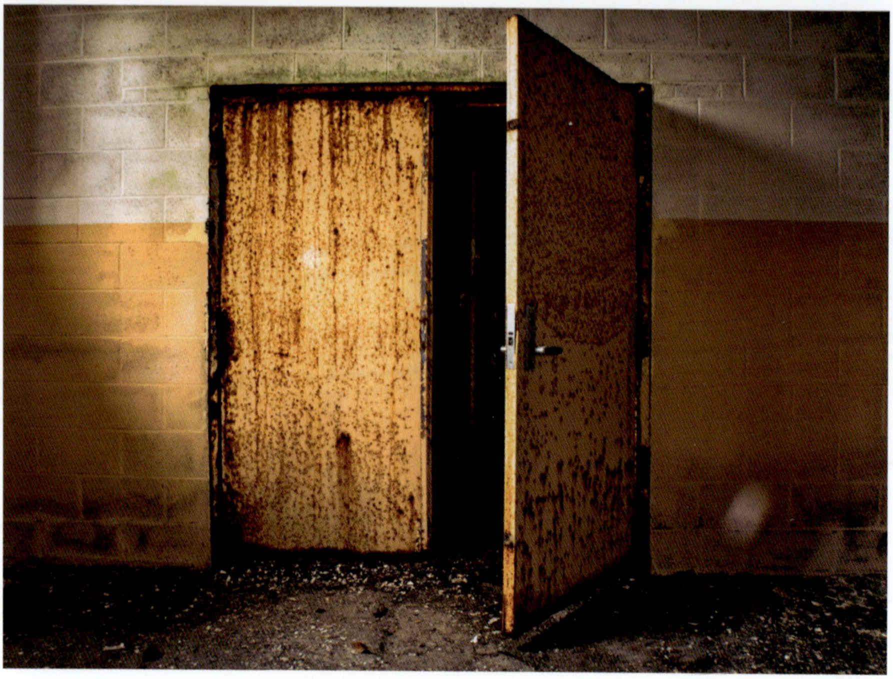

Dark splotches stain the doors with faint faces of the past covering them like tree roots. I don't dare step any further than where her light guides me. My body drifts into the next room. *[Photo by Brian Cray]*

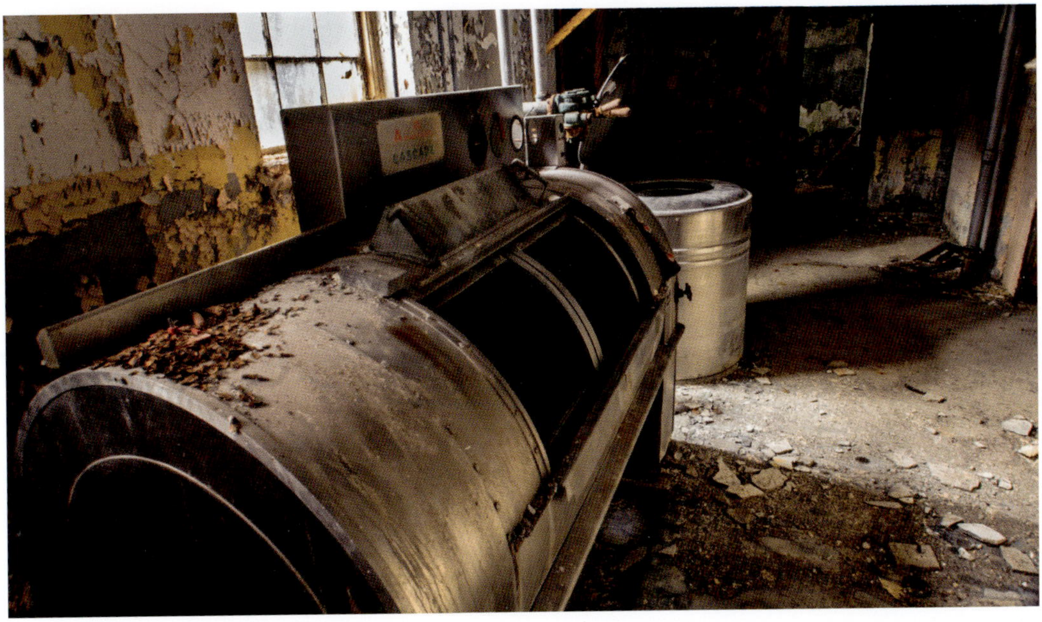

A shuttle of metal gleans under films of decay and I can only wonder what these contraptions did in her heyday? Laundry perhaps? *[Photo by Brian Cray]*

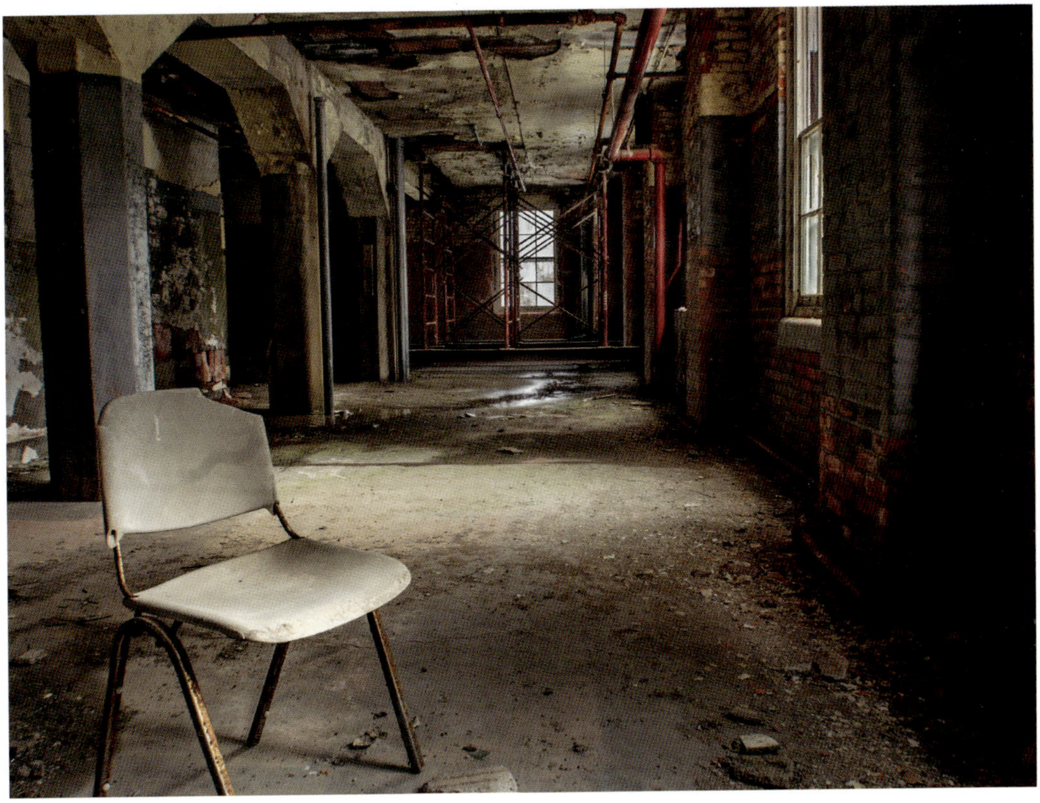

You should grab a copy of Grit-Grin and sit down. This schizophrenic work of random quotes burgeoning with tidbits on tuberculosis establishes a family appeal, treating “the San” like the Brady Bunch. *[Photo by Brian Cray]*

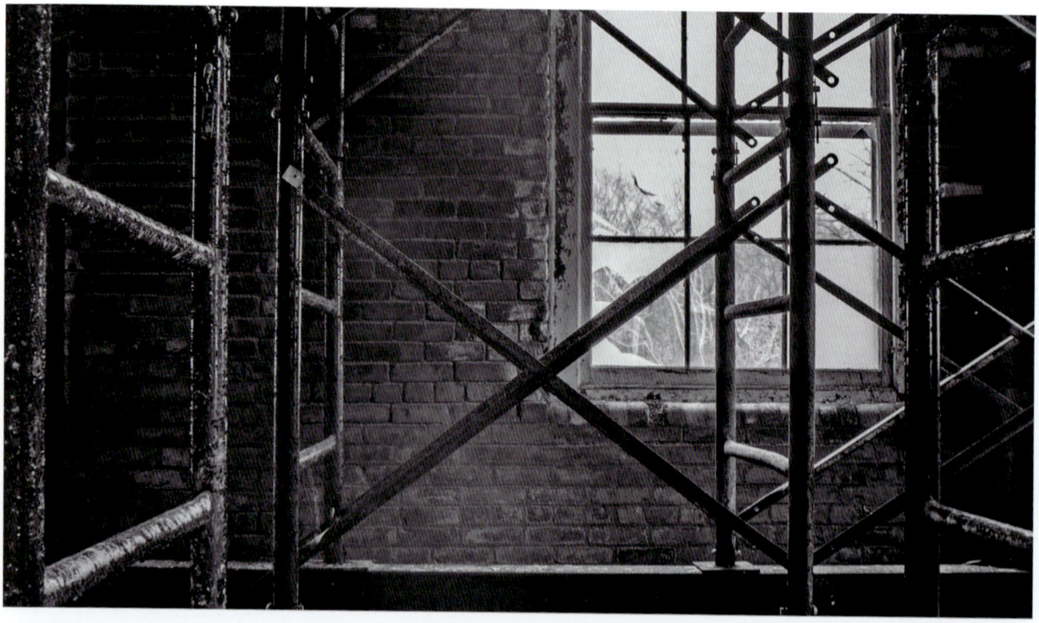

Despite never making it on the National Historic Register these support trusses show that someone once cared about her well-being enough to try to preserve her future. *[Photo by Brian Cray]*

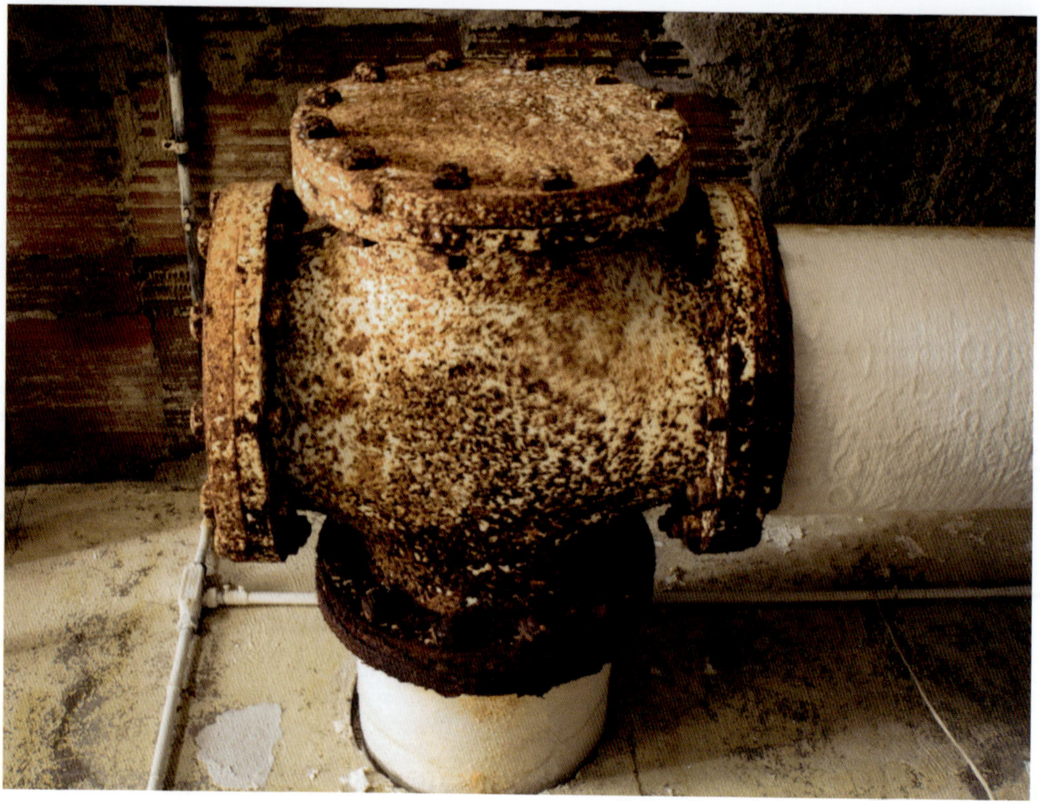

I peek up at the massive trunks of piping. My eyes lock onto a corroded galvanized fitting, so huge it looks like it came off of a cargo ship. *[Photo by Brian Cray]*

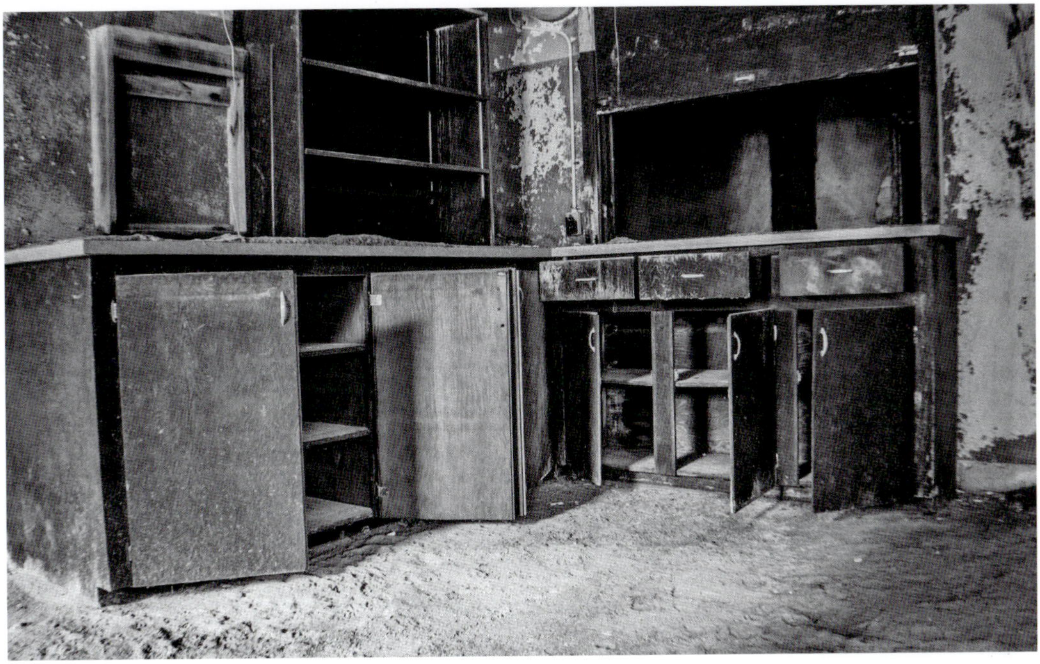

Beneath the massive piping I see the shell of old cabinets. The stale smell of dust and wet countertops permeates my nostrils and I continue onward taking in every piece of decay. *[Photo by Brian Cray]*

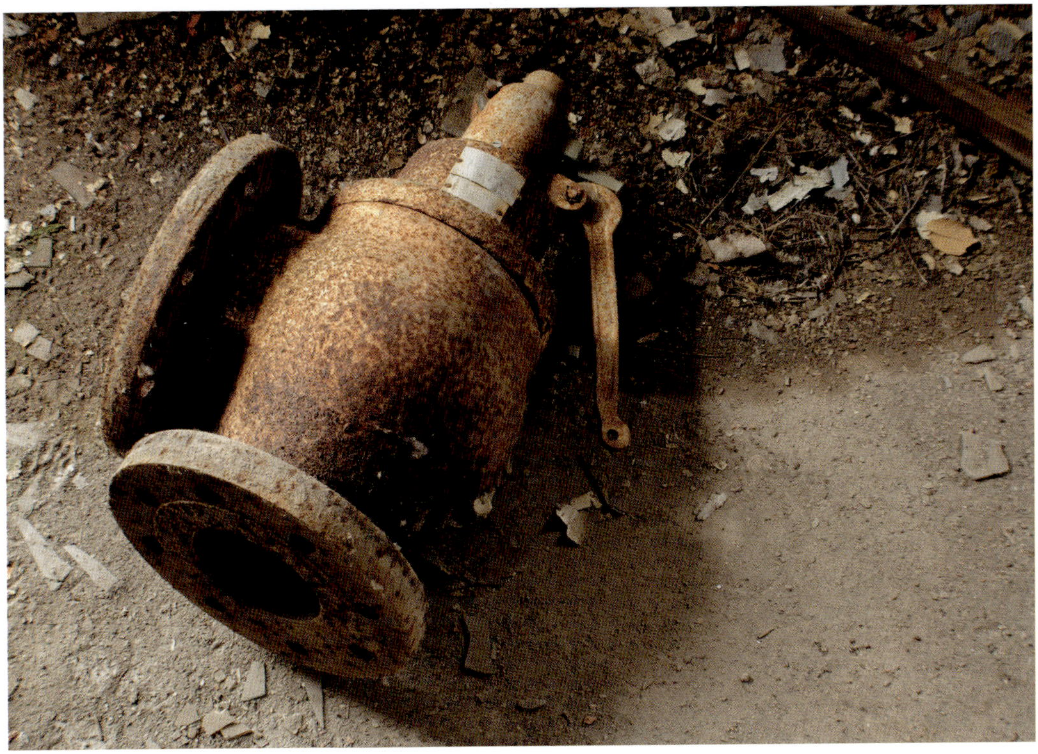

As I trek through ruins it is not uncommon to stumble across loose pipe fittings completely corroded to oblivion. *[Photo by Brian Cray]*

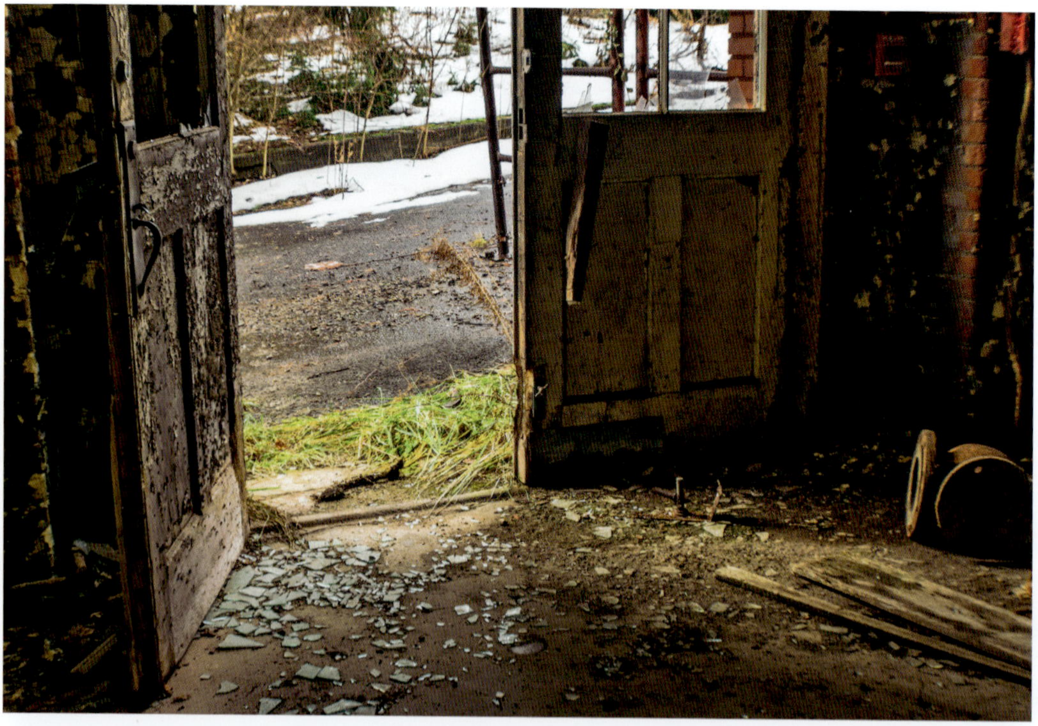

Beyond her decay the vivacious plants fill her scars as nature reclaims its land. Such is the story for most sanitaria across America. *[Photo by Brian Cray]*

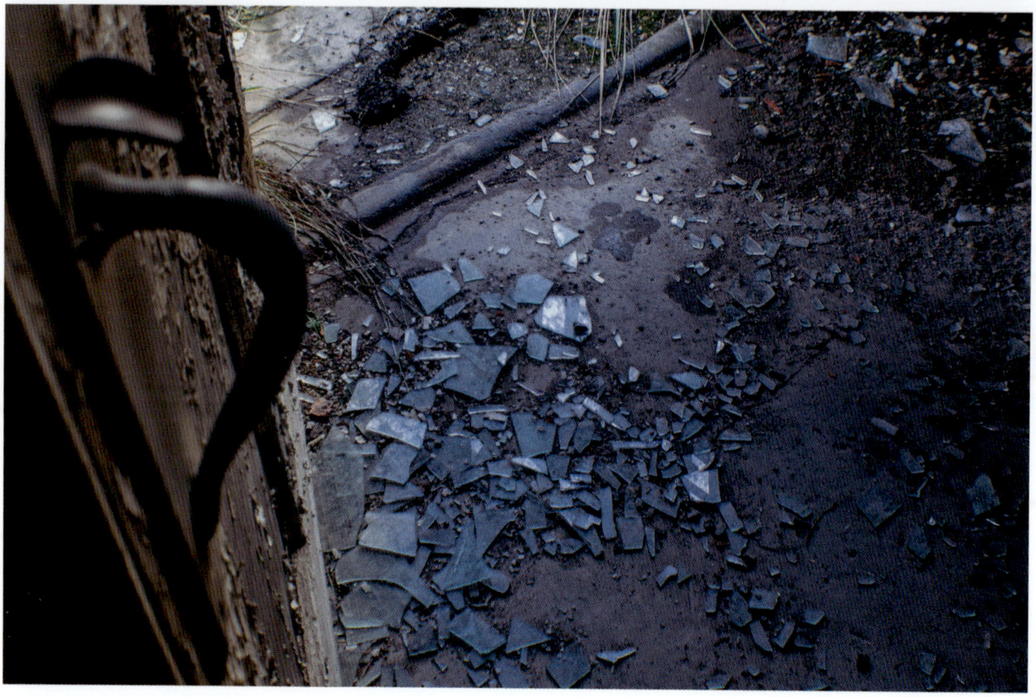

Her frozen reflection strewn in jagged chips of glass across the chilling floor is a common theme throughout each ward and corridor. *[Photo by Brian Cray]*

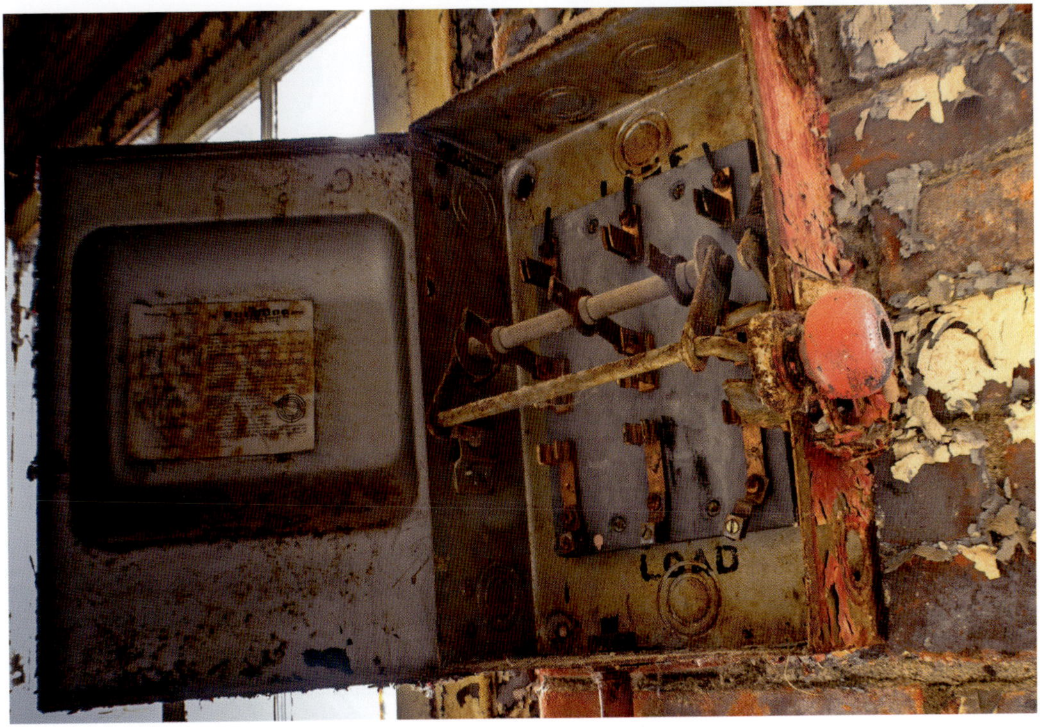

"Bulldog" specializes in security systems and although time sabotaged her wiring system long ago, I can only wonder what this latch once controlled. *[Photo by Brian Cray]*

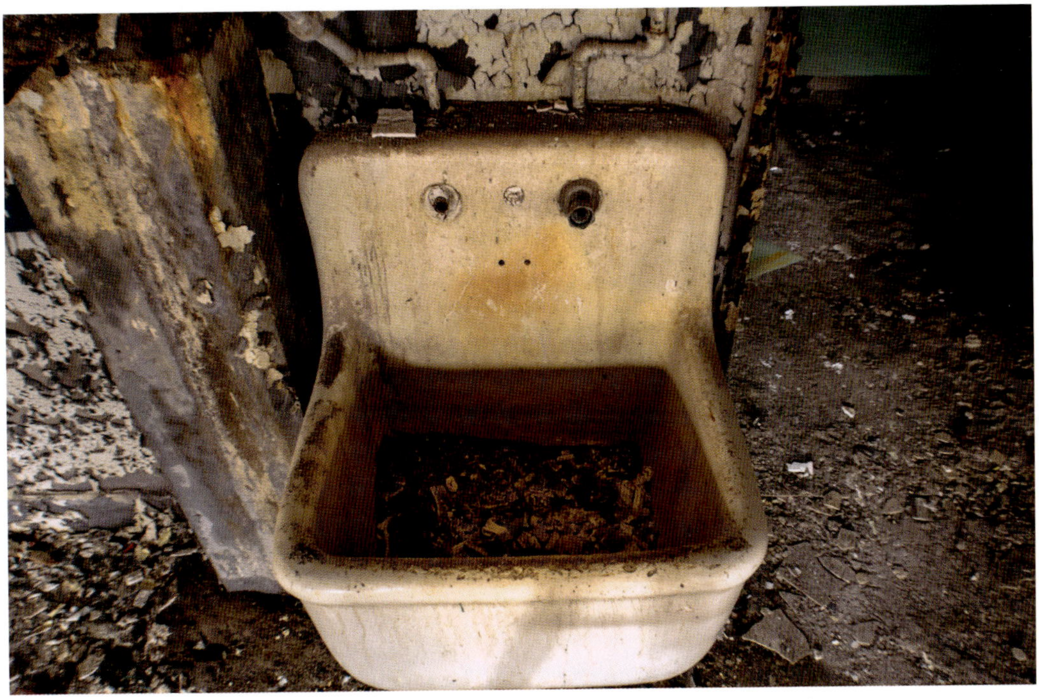

Basic sanitary practices like washing your hands prevented the spread of disease, but did not prevent the spread of tuberculosis, which is an airborne pathogen. *[Photo by Brian Cray]*

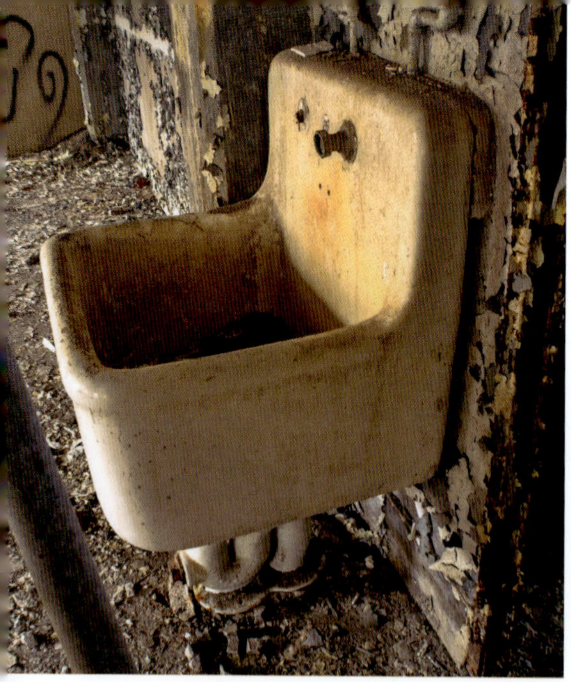

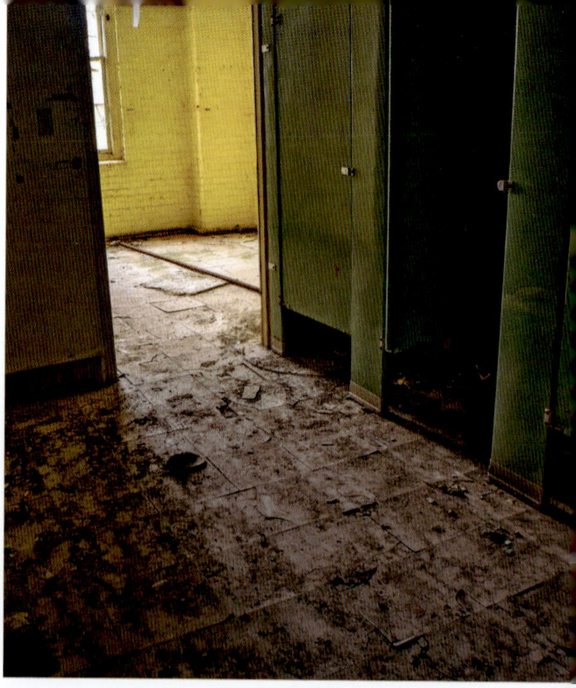

Above left: Pipes hang from the ceiling like dead tree branches. Scabs of paint fester along the floor. The smell of damp tennis shoes permeates the room. I should stop breathing in this muck, but I want to see what lies beyond the tarnished porcelain sink. *[Photo by Brian Cray]*

Above right: As I creep in the shadows of ruin, crumbs of brick and paint chips crunch underfoot and I let out a short yawp. Trembling punches hit my chest as my eyes wander under the bathroom stalls. I think I see a foot, but I'm mistaken. *[Photo by Brian Cray]*

Below left: A flap of paint drapes from the sunflower-yellow wall like a curtain. My eyes drift along the curling tiles and stop at the patterned wallpaper. I wonder if any equipment was left behind. *[Photo by Brian Cray]*

Below right: A large water pipe sprawls out along the floor after plunging from the ceiling. I wonder when they shut off the water. *[Photo by Brian Cray]*

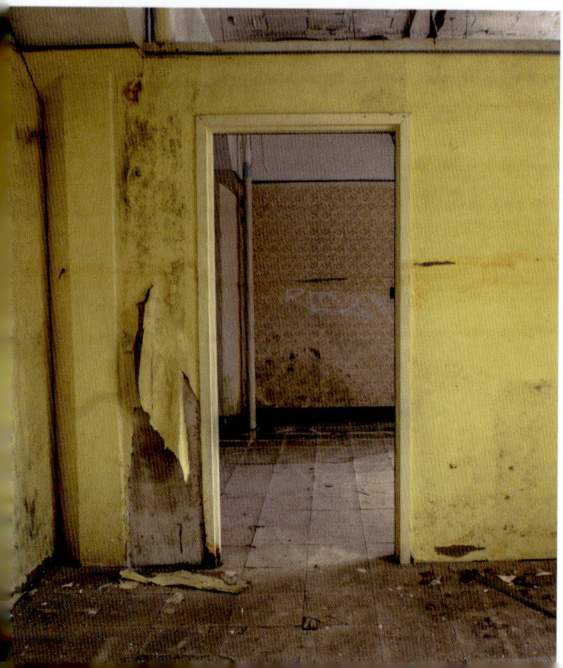

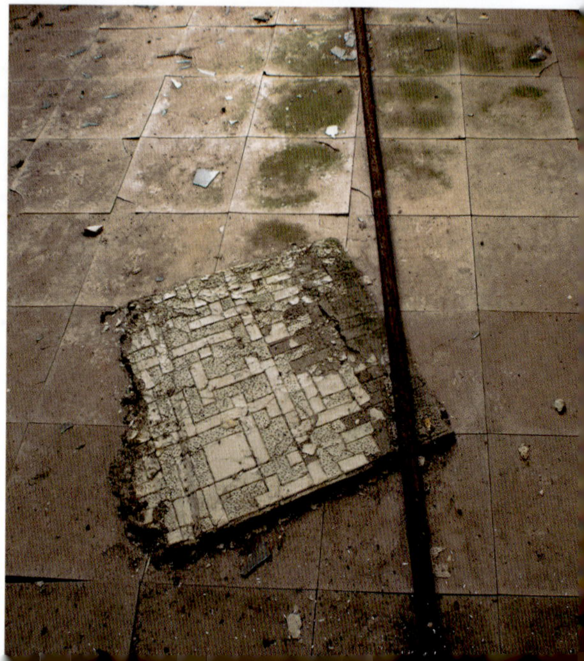

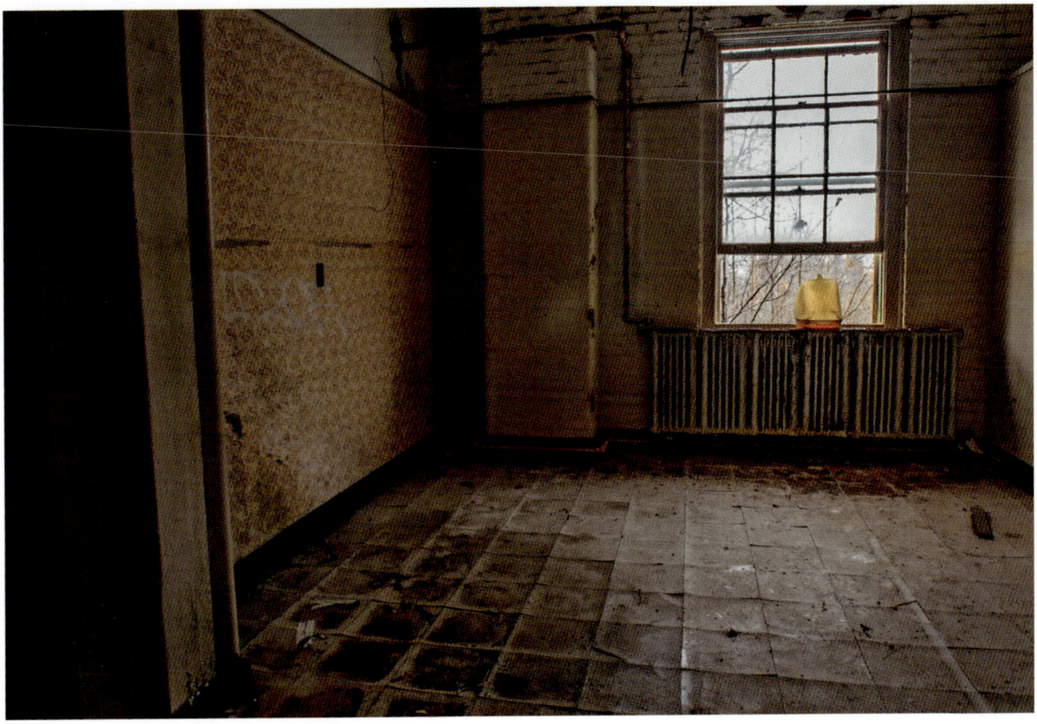

A plastic jug sits atop cavities of a defunct radiator amongst one of the many double hung sash windows. What was this room? *[Photo by Brian Cray]*

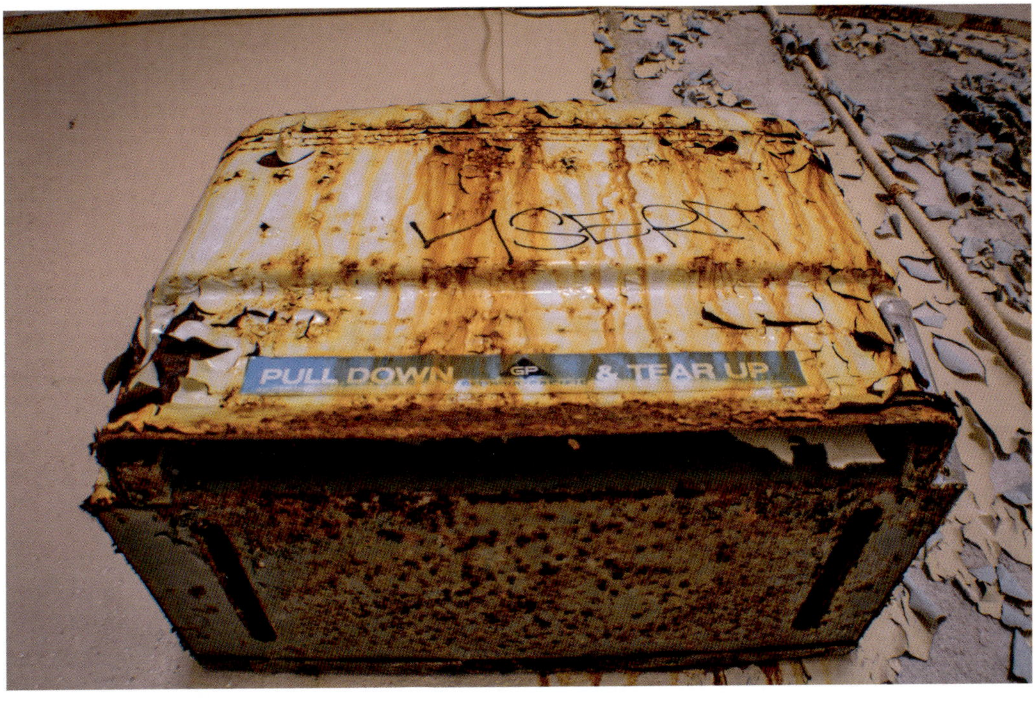

Streaks of sorrow drip down a dispenser of unused toiletries. As I wander deeper through her ruins, it feels esoteric, like the foreshadowing of an apocalypse to come. *[Photo by Brian Cray]*

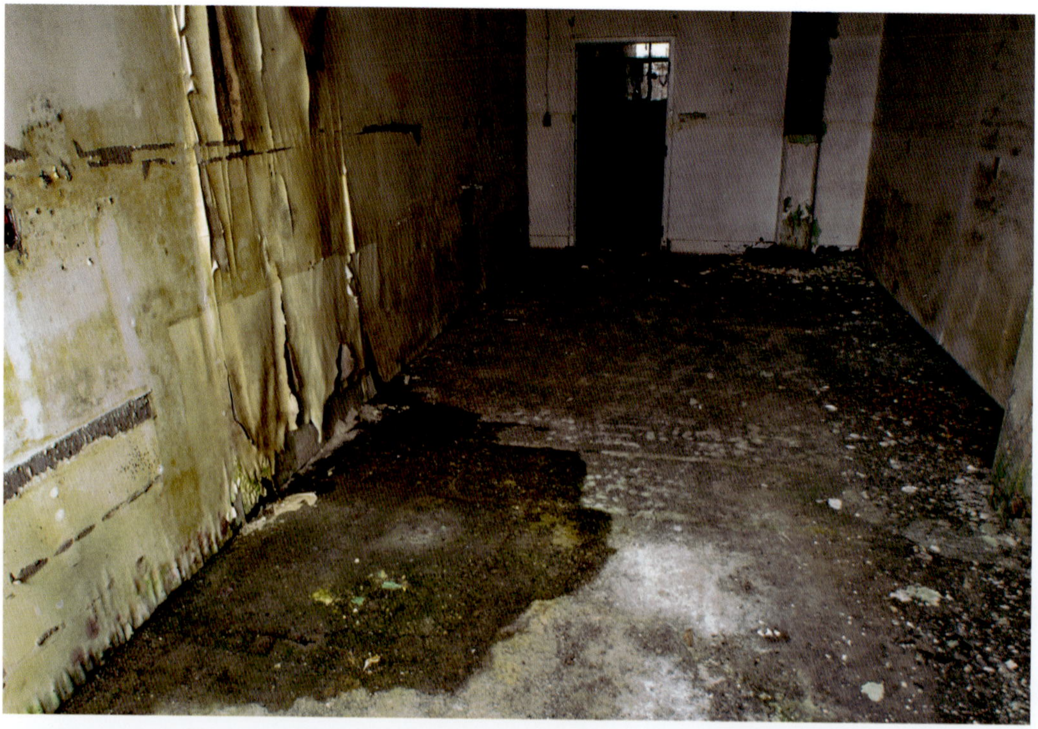

Water bleeds into the floor, tearing through the wall, through gentle drips comprised of many years and tumultuous storms. *[Photo by Brian Cray]*

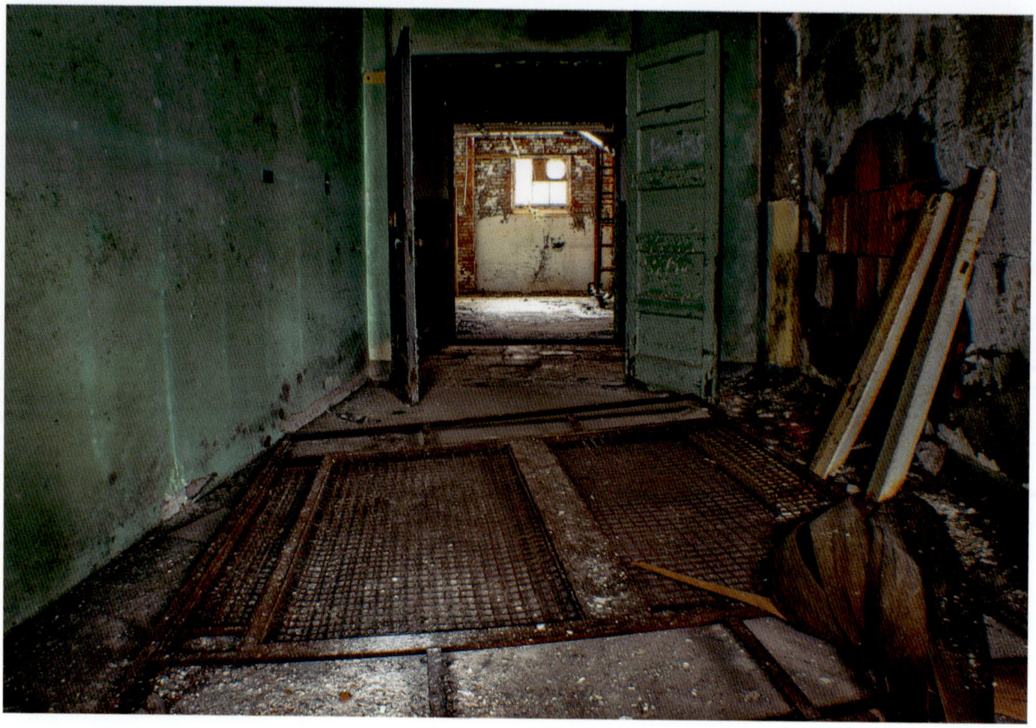

Through every door and windowpane her decay looks the same. *[Photo by Brian Cray]*

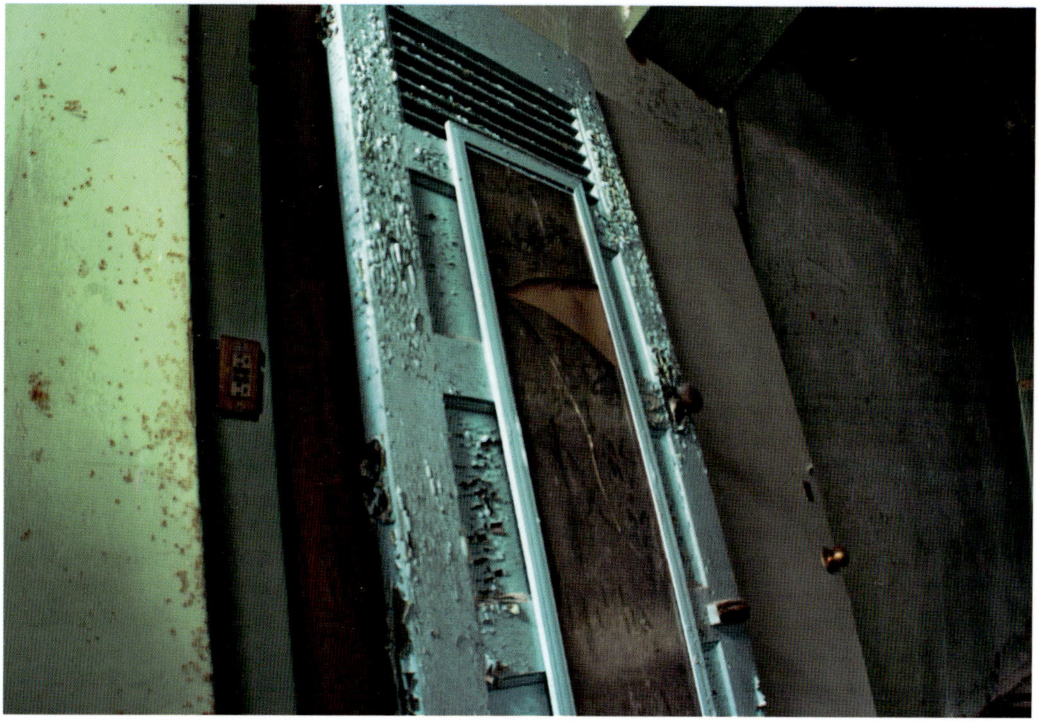

A graveyard of doors stoops along her walls as I glance at a smudged mirror. My reflection is hidden behind its shadow of death. *[Photo by Brian Cray]*

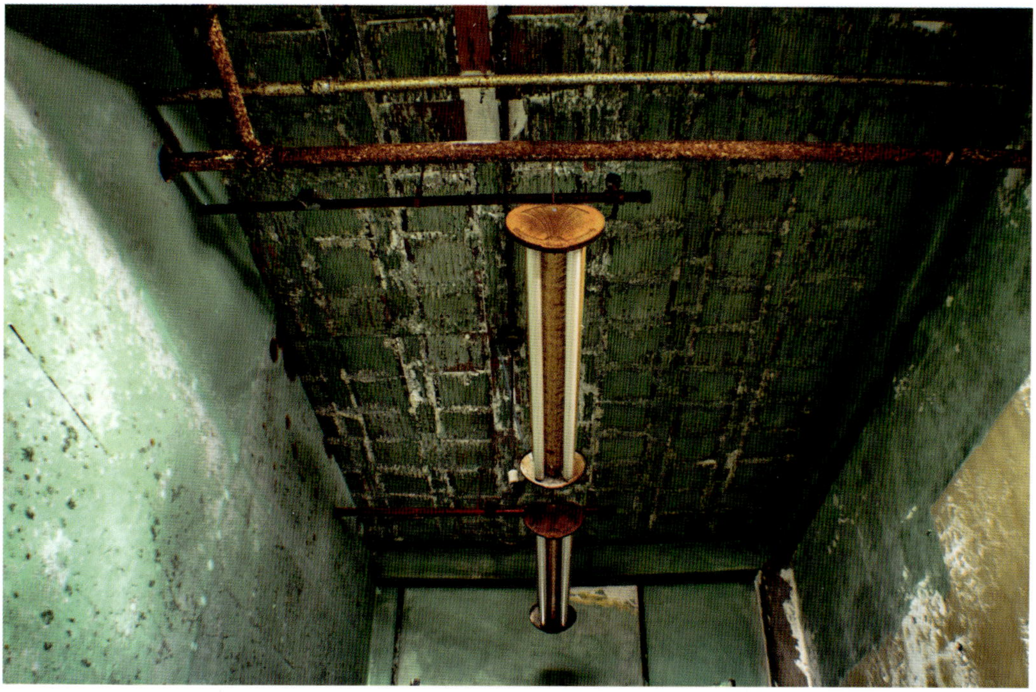

Light fixtures dangle above me on thin puppet strings and I feel like I'm in Dr. Jekyll and Mr. Hyde's laboratory. These walls are unsettling, but maybe it's just my paranoia. *[Photo by Brian Cray]*

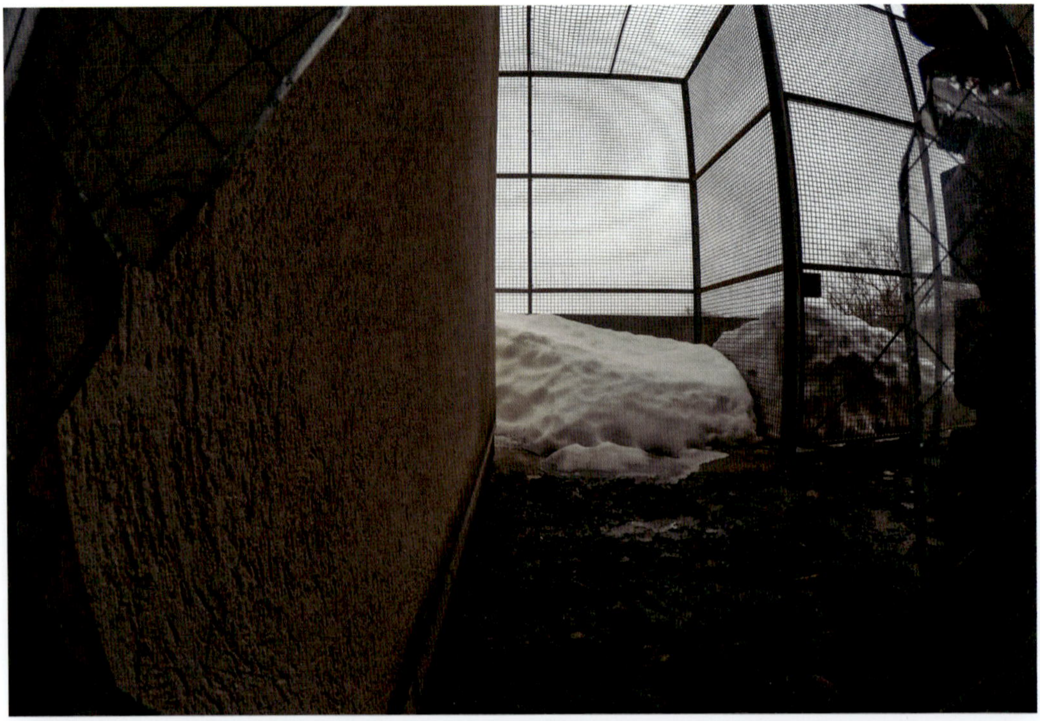

Decomposing leaves decorate the floor like papier-mâché and mud turns to snow. As I break out of my trance, I notice the barricades keeping me in and it feels like a prison. *[Photo by Brian Cray]*

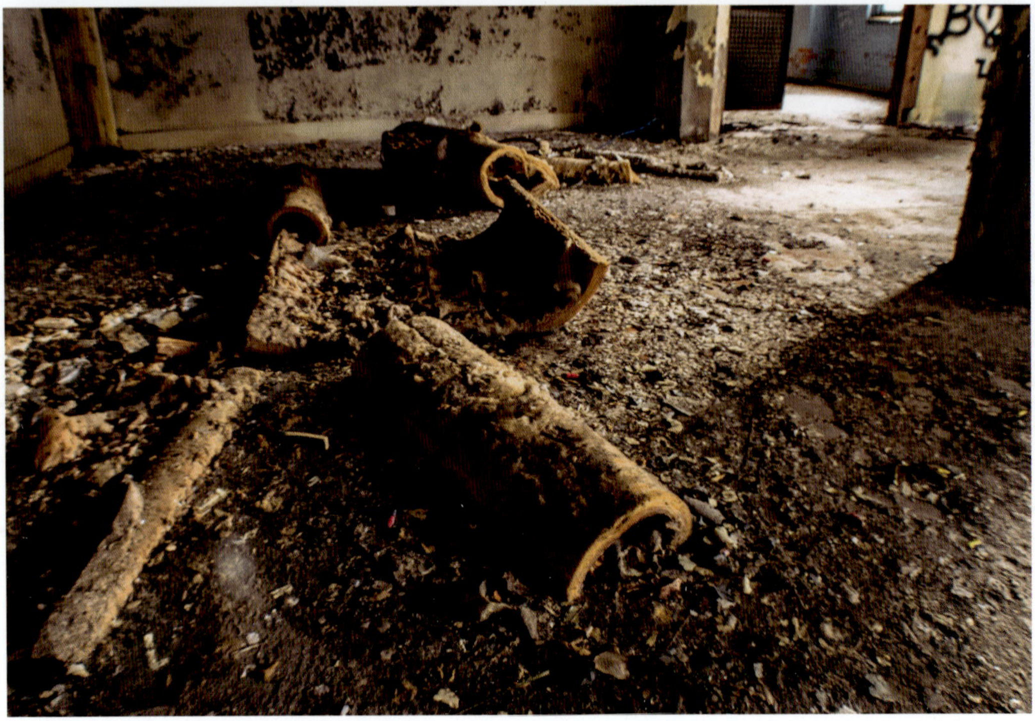

Ductwork coats the floor in patches like feathers from exploded pillows as I follow the radiance. *[Photo by Brian Cray]*

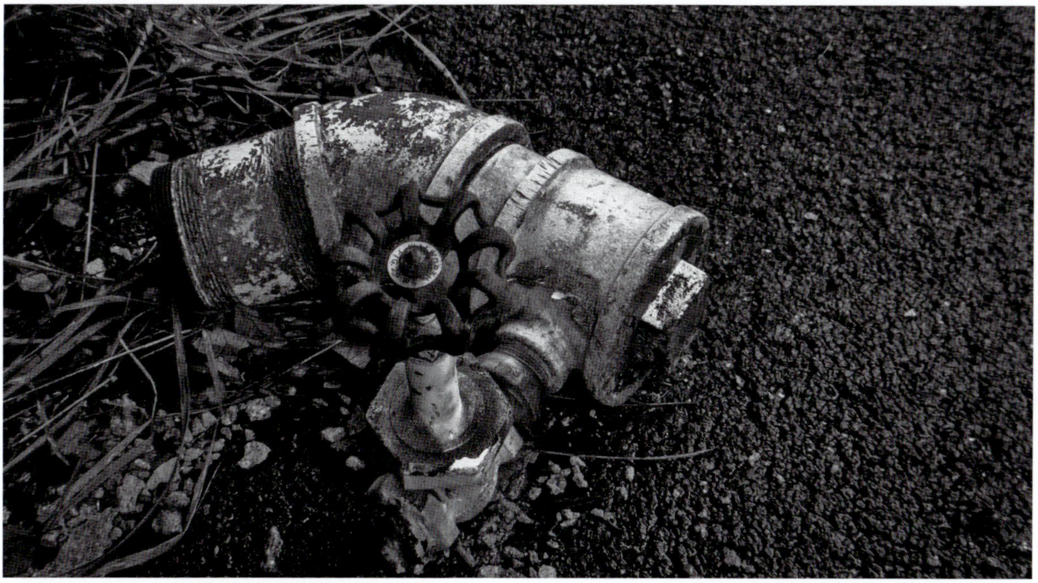

Above: Gate valves run plentiful throughout the complex among the many scattered pieces to her broken heart. *[Photo by Brian Cray]*

Below left: Not even turpentine and a fresh can of paint will heal her deep wounds. *[Photo by Brian Cray]*

Below right: Take a seat and look around. Imagine the past heartache and hardships of the children within these walls. Now picture 36 of them zipping around on a Merry-Go-Round, donated by friends of Mayor Schwab, taking turns, smiling, yelling, cheering, and laughing ("Grit-Grin Magazine," 1927). *[Photo by Brian Cray]*

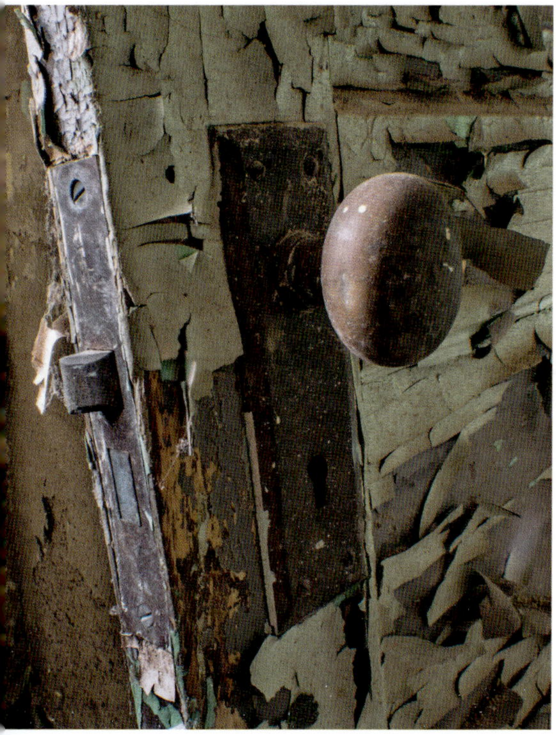

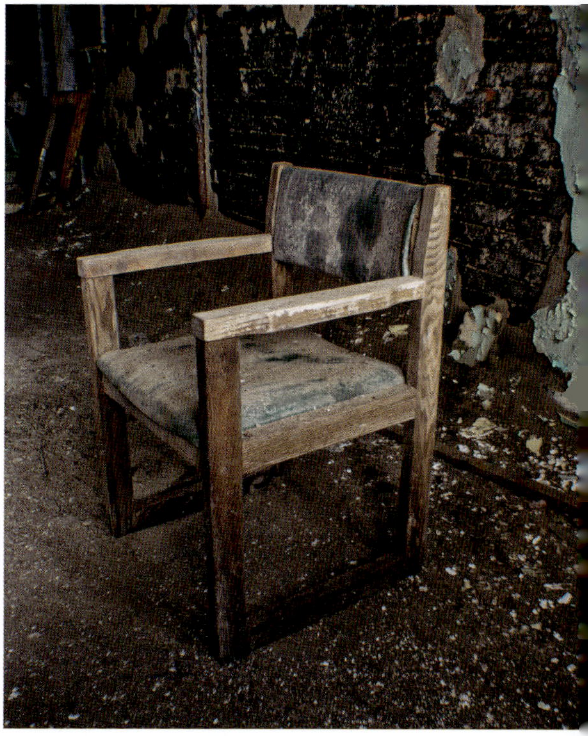

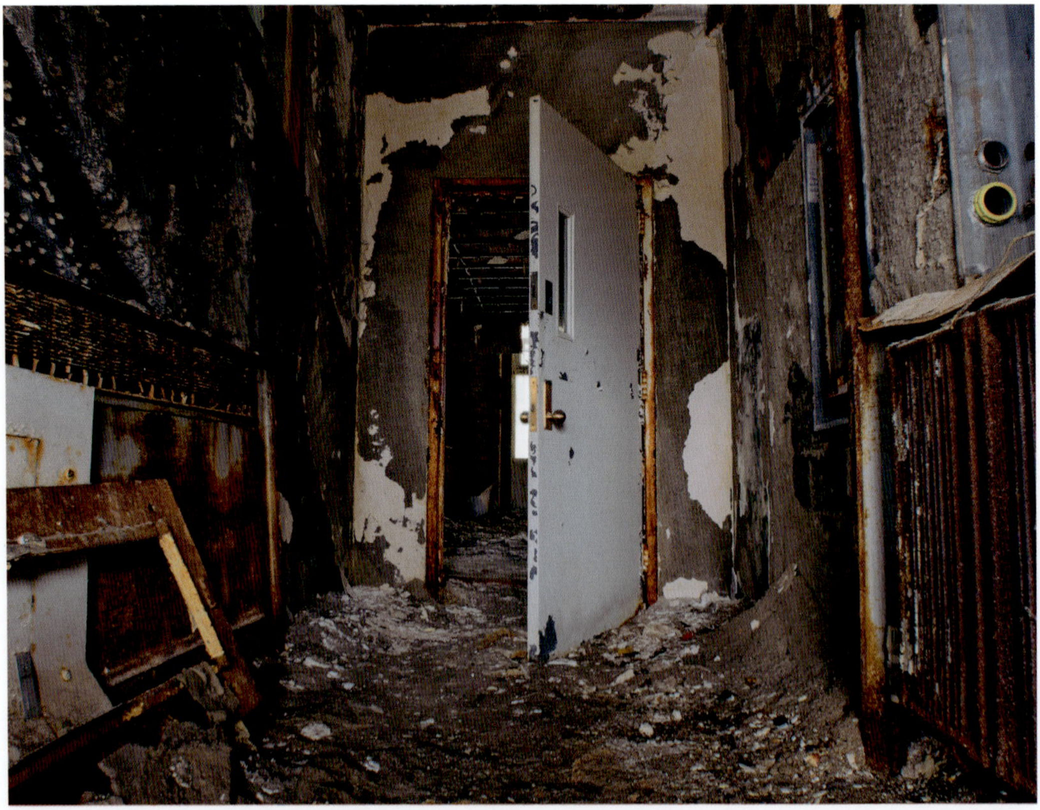

Above: Something about this door feels out of place? *[Photo by Brian Cray]*

Below left: Stories above the ground her ledges crumble at their base as I peer off to the powerhouse beneath the falling sky. *[Photo by Brian Cray]*

Below right: Are the barricades to keep people out or keep patients in? *[Photo by Brian Cray]*

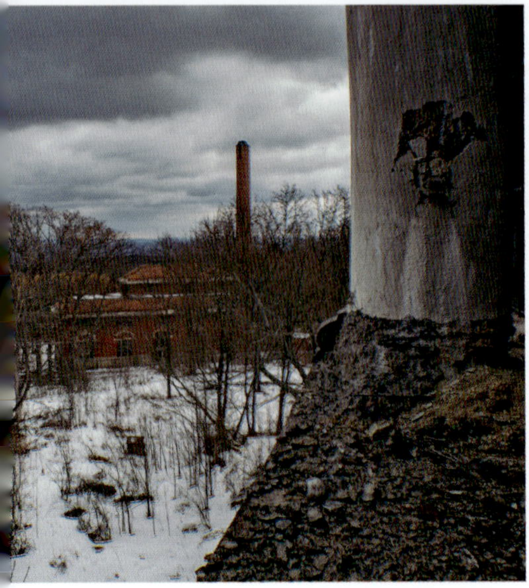

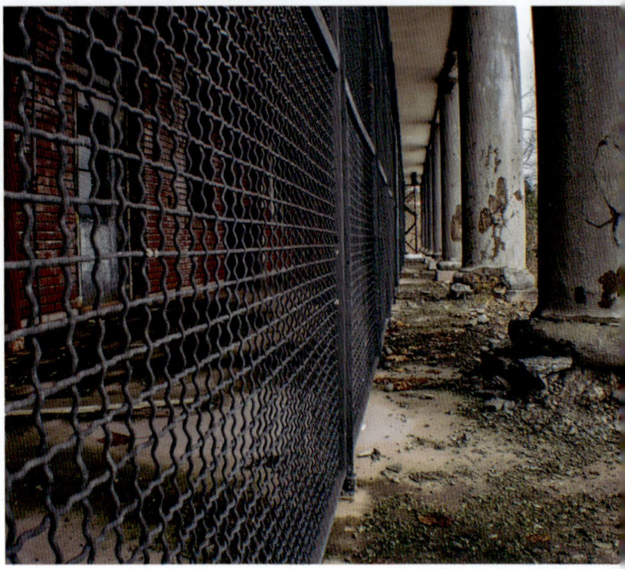

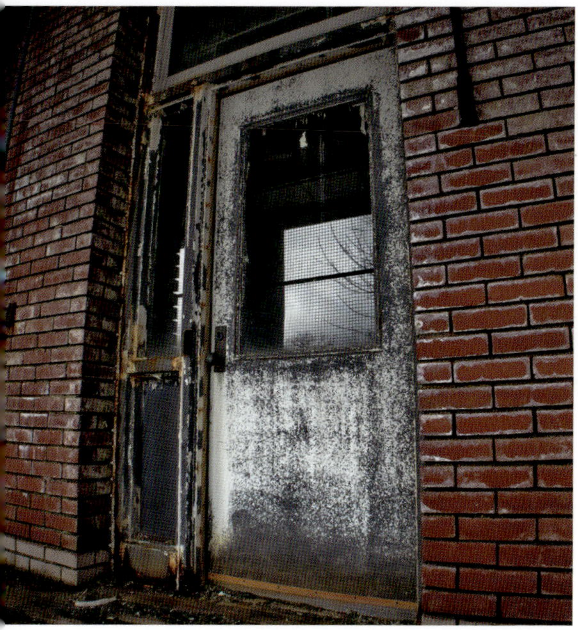

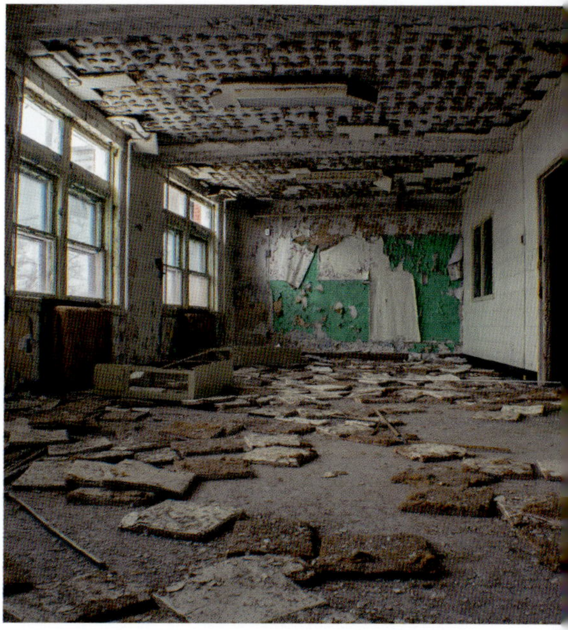

Above left: Looking through one eye is enough to capture her faded smears of decay splotched along every brick and door. *[Photo by Brian Cray]*

Above right: A puzzle paints the floor like a canvas as I wander through the abstract chaos within her morbid walls. *[Photo by Brian Cray]*

Below: Beyond the curving corridors linking Building #2 and Building #1 stands the tallest Christmas tree I have ever seen. I can only hope Christmas cheer helped ease the pain and suffering of those innocent children. *[Photo by Brian Cray]*

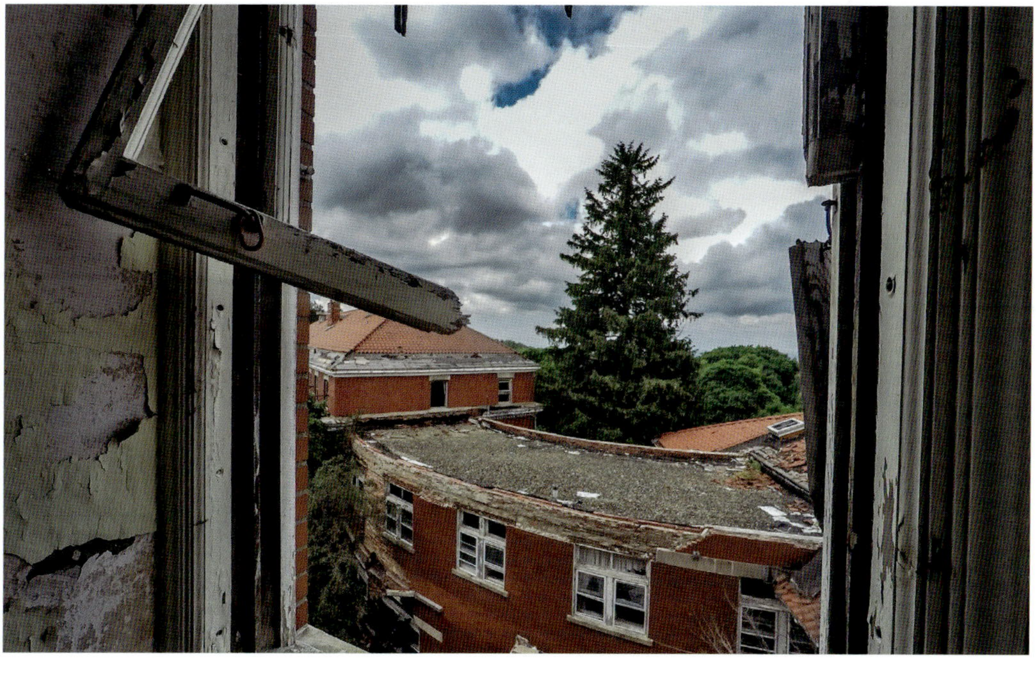

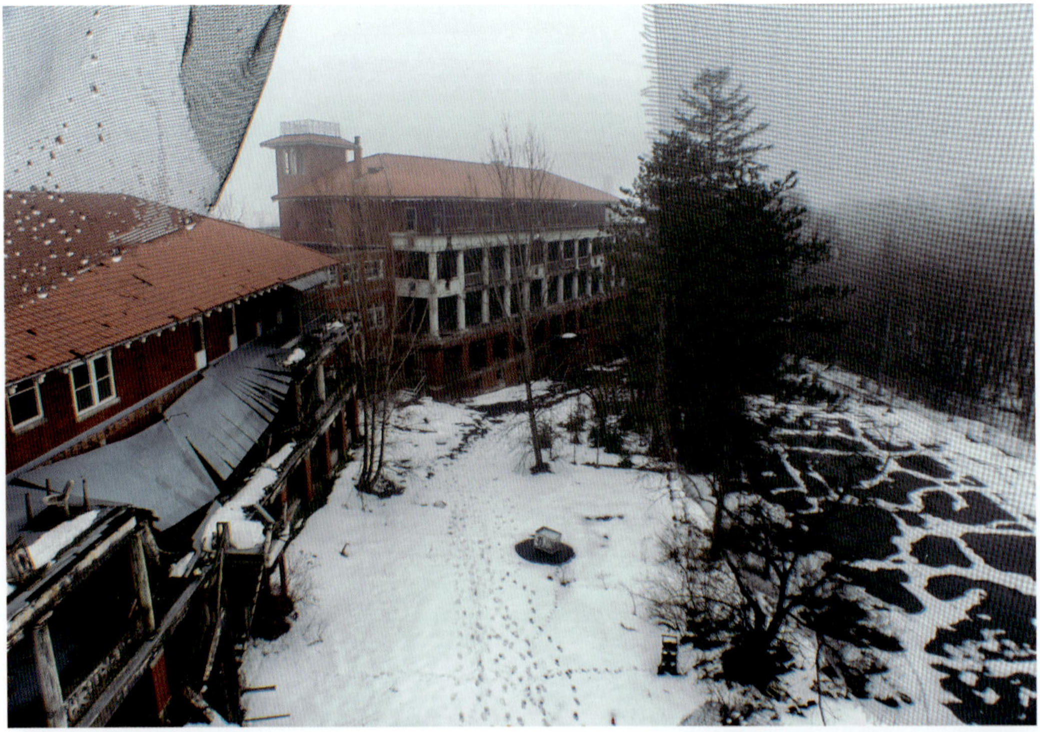

Follow the footprints in the snow and you will find your way through the fencing. *[Photo by Brian Cray]*

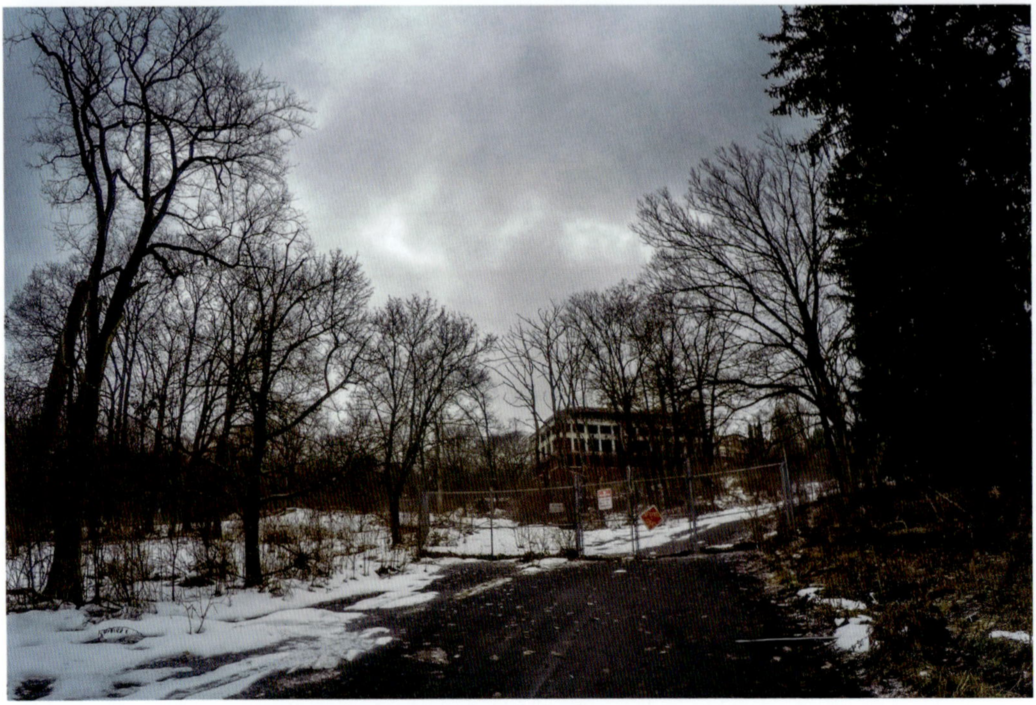

As I turn around, I take one last glance at her legacy before wandering back down Airport Road. I wonder if we will meet again before her last brick falls. *[Photo by Brian Cray]*

APPENDIX A:

J.N. ADAM MEMORIAL HOSPITAL

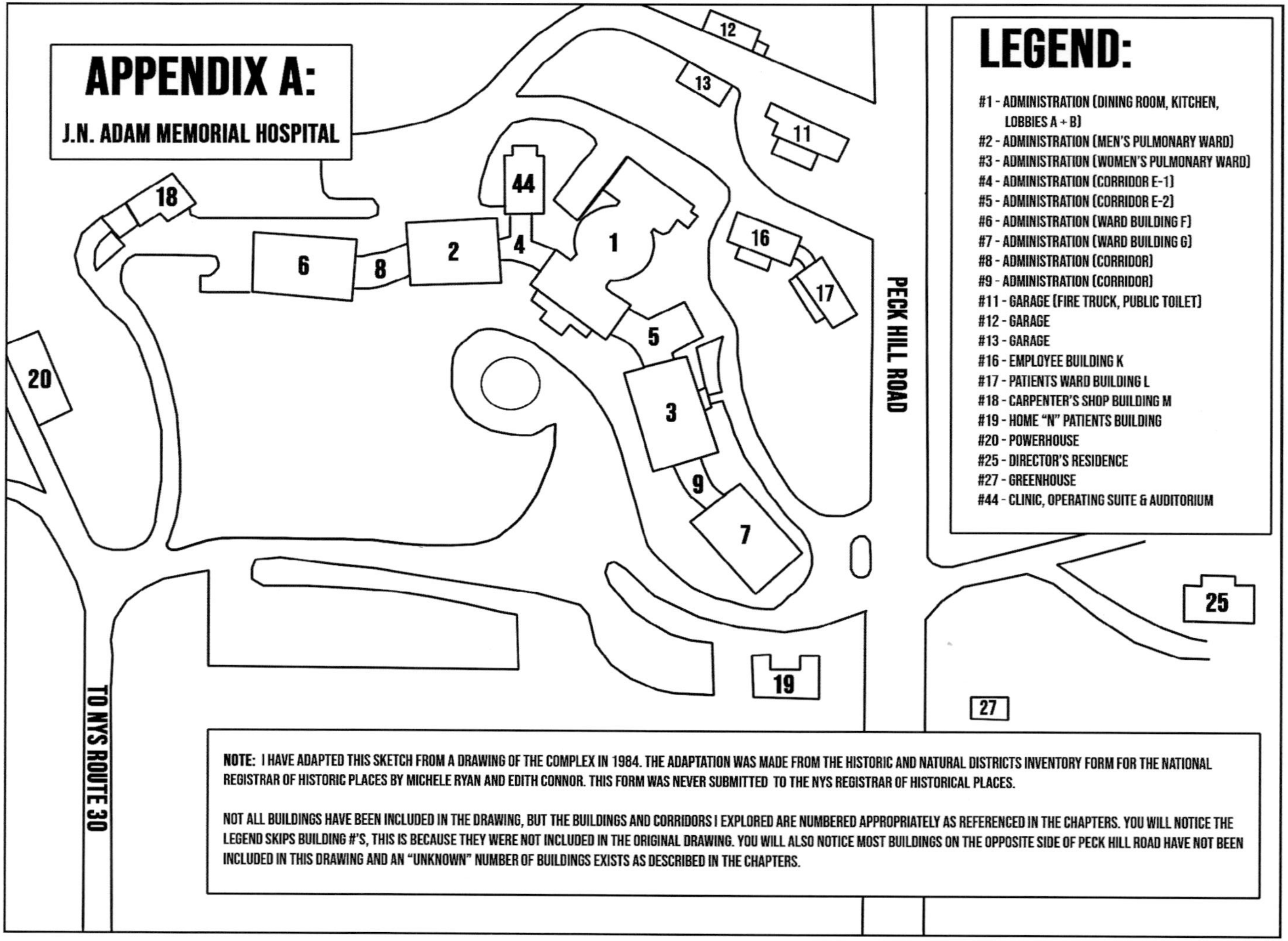

LEGEND:

#1 - ADMINISTRATION (DINING ROOM, KITCHEN, LOBBIES A + B)
#2 - ADMINISTRATION (MEN'S PULMONARY WARD)
#3 - ADMINISTRATION (WOMEN'S PULMONARY WARD)
#4 - ADMINISTRATION (CORRIDOR E-1)
#5 - ADMINISTRATION (CORRIDOR E-2)
#6 - ADMINISTRATION (WARD BUILDING F)
#7 - ADMINISTRATION (WARD BUILDING G)
#8 - ADMINISTRATION (CORRIDOR)
#9 - ADMINISTRATION (CORRIDOR)
#11 - GARAGE (FIRE TRUCK, PUBLIC TOILET)
#12 - GARAGE
#13 - GARAGE
#16 - EMPLOYEE BUILDING K
#17 - PATIENTS WARD BUILDING L
#18 - CARPENTER'S SHOP BUILDING M
#19 - HOME "N" PATIENTS BUILDING
#20 - POWERHOUSE
#25 - DIRECTOR'S RESIDENCE
#27 - GREENHOUSE
#44 - CLINIC, OPERATING SUITE & AUDITORIUM

NOTE: I HAVE ADAPTED THIS SKETCH FROM A DRAWING OF THE COMPLEX IN 1984. THE ADAPTATION WAS MADE FROM THE HISTORIC AND NATURAL DISTRICTS INVENTORY FORM FOR THE NATIONAL REGISTRAR OF HISTORIC PLACES BY MICHELE RYAN AND EDITH CONNOR. THIS FORM WAS NEVER SUBMITTED TO THE NYS REGISTRAR OF HISTORICAL PLACES.

NOT ALL BUILDINGS HAVE BEEN INCLUDED IN THE DRAWING, BUT THE BUILDINGS AND CORRIDORS I EXPLORED ARE NUMBERED APPROPRIATELY AS REFERENCED IN THE CHAPTERS. YOU WILL NOTICE THE LEGEND SKIPS BUILDING #'S, THIS IS BECAUSE THEY WERE NOT INCLUDED IN THE ORIGINAL DRAWING. YOU WILL ALSO NOTICE MOST BUILDINGS ON THE OPPOSITE SIDE OF PECK HILL ROAD HAVE NOT BEEN INCLUDED IN THIS DRAWING AND AN "UNKNOWN" NUMBER OF BUILDINGS EXISTS AS DESCRIBED IN THE CHAPTERS.

ENDNOTES

CHAPTER 1

1 "Perrysburg (town), New York"
2 "Perrysburg (CDP), New York," 2018
3 "Perrysburg, New York"
4 ibid
5 ibid
6 Szabo-Perricelli, 2016
7 "History World TB Day"
8 ibid
9 Shure, 2015
10 Achkar & Jenny-Avital
11 "Timeline," 2015
12 Adams, 2010
13 Szabo-Perricelli, 2016
14 "History World TB Day"
15 ibid
16 Barberis, Bragazzi, Galluzzo, & Martini, 2017
17 "Health in America"
18 Stillman, 1920
19 "Topics in Chronicling America"
20 Rouse, 2018
21 "Mortality Statistics," 1909
22 ibid
23 "A Neighborhood's Continuing Evolution," 2013
24 ibid
25 This whole last paragraph talks about recommended treatments by scientists involving chlorination to prevent the spread of TB, as well as individual studies showing active TB

due to subpar sanitation standards all sourced from Greenberg, 1957 in *Tuberculosis Transmission by Waste Waters: A Review. Sewage and Industrial Wastes.*

26 "Trends in Mortality"

27 "Vaccines Basic TB Facts"

CHAPTER 2

1 Dunster, et al., 1917

2 ibid

3 ibid

4 ibid

5 ibid

6 LoGrasso, 1921

7 Bendes, 1922

8 In regard to Dr. Rollier's percentage of cured patients in Leysin, Switzerland, the number seems too high to be believable, so this statistical data should be taken lightly, too. There was a lot of dishonesty in the early 1900s surrounding alternative medical practices and their validity.

9 Dunster, et. al., 1917; LoGrasso, 1921

10 LoGrasso, 1921

11 LoGrasso, 1921; Bendes, 1922

12,13 These excerpts were interpolated from three sources, one written by Dr. Bendes from a 1922 publication in the *Journal Lancet,* the other from LoGrasso in a 1921 publication in *Health News* and the last from Hyde and LoGrasso in a 1917 publication in *New York Medical Journal.* All three of them worked at the J. N. Adam Memorial Hospital so there is bias as to whether or not heliotherapy was effective at all.

14 Dunster, et al., 1917

15 "Perrysburg Sun Cure," 1919

16 Dunster, et al., 1917

17 Fitzgerald, 1926

18 Szabo-Perricelli, 2016

19 "Perrysburg Sun Cure," 1919

20 *Grit and Grin* was a magazine published by the J. N. Adam Memorial Hospital making a lot of the allegations about the effectiveness of the sun cure quite biased.

21 Fitzgerald, 1926

22 ibid

23 ibid

24 Ruslander, 1920

25 ibid

26 ibid

27, 28, 30, 31, 33, 35, 37 My interpolations of the intentions of the hospital are a mixed bag. Part of me would like to believe that such a utopian sanitarium existed to foster resistance against tuberculosis and solidify "honest" research of heliotherapy against this terminal illness. But, my other half bodes towards the potential cases of neglect and abuse that went undocumented, as well as dishonest practices and falsifying the effectiveness of treatments through skewed statistical data. I'm sure many patients experienced both positive and negative treatment and I would presume they'd be hard-pressed to divulge such information after all these years. This is all my opinion based from anonymous quotes and one story read from Char Szabo-Perricelli's *Her Inside Voice* and through email correspondence with the town historian, Jody Shaw. In Jody's personal experience, none of these horror stories were ever divulged to her, as people had nothing but standing ovations towards the hospital, but more than one instance of mistreatment could have existed. Jody also mentioned a man who stayed in an adjacent ward while his mother was being treated for tuberculosis at the sanitarium. Once his mother died, they released him as "cured," even though he never had TB.

29 Szabo-Perricelli, 2016

33 Dunster, et al., 1917

34 Szabo-Perricelli

36 Epstein, 2003

CHAPTER 3

1 Hamilton, 1906

2 Szabo-Perricelli, 2016

3 Fitzgerald, 1926

4 Szabo-Perricelli, 2016

5 Fitzgerald, 1926

6 Dalkowski, 2017

7 Szabo-Perricelli, 2016

8 Dalkowski, 2017; Dunster, et al., 1917

9 Ryan, 1985

10 Dunster, et al., 1917; Ryan, 1985

11 This number may not be accurate. It was taken from the yellow inventory form Doc. No. 915D00047, which states there are fifty-seven buildings, but in the figures it shows fifty-nine, so it is off by an unknown amount of buildings. I could not verify from other sources the total number of structures on-site, but I believe it is somewhere between forty-four and fifty-seven.

12 Ryan, 1985

13 Dalkowski, 2017; Ryan, 1985

14 Ryan, 1985

15 ibid

16,17, 18, 19, 20, 21 Buildings #1, #2, #3, #6, #7, #18, #20 and #44 along with the connecting corridors are mentioned because those were the buildings I explored and took photographs of, which you will see in the following pages. Refer to Appendix A to see their locations. Information was interpolated from a 2017 appraisal written by John A. Dalkowski, and a yellow Historic and Natural Districts Inventory form (Doc. No. 915D00047) from 1985 submitted by Michele Ryan.

22 Dalkowski, 2017; Ryan, 1985

23 "Perrysburg Campus Property," 1989

24 Dalkowski, 2017
25 Dalkowski, 2017; Szabo-Perricelli, 2016
26 "Perrysburg Campus Property," 1989
27 Dalkowski, 2017
28 "Friends of J. N. Adam Historic Landmark & Forest," 2014
29 Dalkowski, 2017
30 "Friends of J. N. Adam Historic Landmark & Forest," 2014
31 Dalkowski, 2017
32 Benjamin, 2005
33 Dalkowski, 2017
34 ibid
35 "J N Adam Facility"

BIBLIOGRAPHY

(n.d.). Retrieved January 18, 2018, from http://www1.nyc.gov/html/dep/html/drinking_water/history.shtml

(n.d.). Retrieved January 15, 2019, from https://assembly.state.ny.us/leg/?default_fld=&bn=A7145&term=2015&Memo=Y

Doc. No. 915D00047, (1984). Historic and Natural Districts Inventory form for the National Registrar of Historic Places written by Michele Ryan and/or Edith Connor

Achievements in Public Health, 1900-1999: Safer and Healthier Foods. (n.d.). Retrieved February 03, 2019, from https://www.cdc.gov/mmwr/preview/mmwrhtml/mm4840a1.htm

Achkar, J. M., & Jenny-Avital, E. R. (n.d.). Incipient and Subclinical Tuberculosis: Defining Early ... Retrieved February 9, 2019, from https://www.ncbi.nlm.nih.gov/pmc/articles/PMC3192549/

Adams, M. (2010). *Mr. America: How muscular millionaire Bernarr Macfadden transformed the nation through sex, salad, and the ultimate starvation diet.* United States: It Books.

Barberis, I., Bragazzi, N. L., Galluzzo, L., & Martini, M. (2017, March). The history of tuberculosis: From the first historical records to the isolation of Koch's bacillus. Retrieved January 3, 2019, from https://www.ncbi.nlm.nih.gov/pubmed/28515626/

Beahan, L. (2005). J. N. Adam Memorial Hospital Buffalo's Tuberculosis Sanatorium at PERRYSBURG. 1-8. doi:https://niagarasierraclub.files.wordpress.com/2011/05/perrysburgarticle_behan.pdf&ved=2ahUKEwiSpZPStq_gAhWI11kKHbStDNIQFjAMegQIAhAB&usg=AOvVaw1tmQG88GNApVXfnJg7-0WW

Bendes, J.H. (1922). *The Journal-lancet* (Vol. 42). Lancet Publications. doi:https://play.google.com/store/books/details?id=_tYyAQAAMAAJ

Benjamin, E. (2005, July 8). Last Gasp for Hospital? Retrieved February 9, 2019, from https://web.archive.org/web/20070211072535/http://www.nationaltrust.org/magazine/archives/arch_story/070805.htm

Budds, D. (2018, October 02). How microbes 'designed' New York. Retrieved January 15, 2019, from https://ny.curbed.com/2018/10/2/17925378/nyc-museum-exhibit-germs-public-housing

Cichon, S., & Cichon, S. (2016, November 28). Buffalo in the '20s: At JN Adam Memorial, a groundbreaking 'sun cure' for tuberculosis. Retrieved December 19, 2018, from https://buffalonews.com/2016/11/28/buffalo-20s-sun-cure-tuberculosis/

Croyle, J., & Croyle, J. (2018, May 23). Cholera, smallpox, scarlet fever: Epidemics that swept through 19th Century Syracuse. Retrieved November 30, 2018, from https://www.syracuse.com/vintage/2018/05/cholera_smallpox_scarlet_fever_syracuse_faced_epidemics_throughout_19th_century.html

Dalkowski, J. A. (2017). *A Marketing Study and Strategic Plan as of October 18, 2016* (pp. 1-371, Rep.). National Real Estate Research, LLC. doi:https://ogs.ny.gov/bu/dc/docs/2017/National_Appraisal_Report.pdf&ved=2ahUKEwihguHno6_gAhUEON8KHY-YAKMQFjAQegQICBAB&usg=AOvVaw1ZZxLKjpkURUyEQKw_DDmF
An appraisal report for the J. N. Adam Memorial Complex

Doctor Builds Miniature of Adam Hospital. (n.d.). *Buffalo Courier-Express*. Retrieved February 9, 2019, from https://web.archive.org/web/20130309050038/http://jnadam.org/history/1940-0407.pdf. Published April 7, 1940

Early Research and Treatment of Tuberculosis in the 19th Century. (n.d.). Retrieved December 19, 2018, from http://exhibits.hsl.virginia.edu/alav/tuberculosis/

Epstein, R. H. (2003, May 27). A Magic Mountain of Fresh Air, Sexual Frolicking and, Oh, Yes, Recovery. Retrieved February 9, 2019, from https://www.nytimes.com/2003/05/27/health/a-magic-mountain-of-fresh-air-sexual-frolicking-and-oh-yes-recovery.html

Fitzgerald, R. E. (1926). Perrysburg—A Mecca For Heliotherapy. *American Journal of Public Health, 16*(9), 893-895. doi:10.2105/ajph.16.9.893

Friends of J. N. Adam Historic Landmark & Forest. (2014, September 5). Retrieved February 9, 2019, from https://web.archive.org/web/20140905065635/http://jnadam.org/

Greenberg, A., & Kupka, E. (1957). Tuberculosis Transmission by Waste Waters: A Review. *Sewage and Industrial Wastes, 29*(5), 524-537. Retrieved from http://www.jstor.org/stable/25033338

Grit-Grin Magazine August 1927. (n.d.). Retrieved February 9, 2019, from https://cdm16694.contentdm.oclc.org/digital/collection/p16694coll80/id/170/rec/3

Guerrieri, V. (2018, October 10). Underwater Archaeologists May Have Discovered the Oldest Shipwreck in Lake Erie. Retrieved February 28, 2019, from https://smithsonianmag.co/history/underwater-archaeologists-may-have-discovered-oldest-shipwreck-lake-erie-180970503/

Hamilton, T.P. (1906). *World Today* (Vol. 11). Current Encyclopedia Company. doi:https://play.google.com/store/books/details?id=SJjNAAAAMAAJ

History I World TB Day I TB I CDC. (n.d.). Retrieved November 4, 2018, from https://www.cdc.gov/tb/worldtbday/history.htm

Health in America. (n.d.). Retrieved January 15, 2019, from https://www.cuny.edu/site/cc/health-in-america/1900s.html

Hyde, C.L., & LoGrasso, H. (1917). *International Record of Medicine and General Practice Clinics* (Vol. 105) (E.S. Dunster, F.P. Foster, J. Bradbridge, & C. Eucharist, Eds.). MD Publications. doi:https://play.google.com/store/books/details?id=aFFQAQAAMAAJ

J N Adam Facility. (n.d.). Retrieved February 9, 2019, from https://historicpath.com/article/j-n-adam-facility-192

Journal of the Outdoor Life (Vol. 20). (1923). doi:https://play.google.com/store/books/details?id=hbAhAQAAMAAJ

LoGrasso, H. (1921). *Health News*(Vol. 36, Part 16 - 37, Part 17). The Department. doi:https://play.google.com/store/books/details?id=lmrf1pL3XkAC

Mortality Statistics. (1909). U.S. Government Printing Office. doi:https://play.google.com/store/books/details?id=MeQPFMyC51IC
New York State Journal of Medicine(Vol. 15-16). (1915). Medical Society of the State of New York. doi:https://play.google.com/store/books/details?id=x4xMAQAAMAAJ

Nickel city owns a quarter. (n.d.). Retrieved February 01, 2019, from http://www.observertoday.com/news/local-region/2017/10/nickel-city-owns-a-quarter/

Perrysburg Campus Property(pp. 1-10, Rep.). (1989). J. N. Adam Developmental Disabilities Service Office. doi:https://web.archive.org/web/20130310005556/http://jnadam.org/history/PropertySummary1989.pdf

1989 Property Summary of the J. N. Adam Memorial Hospital

Perrysburg (CDP), New York. (2018, July 25). Retrieved February 9, 2019, from https://en.m.wikipedia.org/wiki/Perrysburg_(CDP),_New_York

Perrysburg (town), New York. (2018, November 04). Retrieved February 9, 2019, from https://en.m.wikipedia.org/wiki/Perrysburg_(town),_New_York

Perrysburg, New York. (n.d.). Retrieved February 9, 2019, from https://enchantedmountains.com/community/perrysburg

Perrysburg Sun Cure is Most Effective. (1919). *The Arrow,2*(20). doi:https://web.archive.org/web/20130309050114/http://jnadam.org/history/PierceArrowarticle.pdf

Proceedings of the Common Council of the City of Buffalo. (1919). The Council. doi:https://play.google.com/store/books/details?id=wPNHAQAAMAAJ

Rouse, K. L. (2018, June 23). Meat Inspection Act of 1906. Retrieved February 01, 2019, from https://www.britannica.com/topic/Meat-Inspection-Act

Shure, N. (2015, March 23). How New York Beat Its TB Epidemic. Retrieved December 29, 2018, from https://www.thedailybeast.com/how-new-york-beat-its-tb-epidemic

Siegmund, W. P. (n.d.). Read "Memorial Tributes: Volume 7" at NAP.edu. Retrieved February 9, 2019, from https://nap.edu/4779/chapter/33

Stillman, E. G. (1920). *Hospital Social Service* (Vol. 2). New York, NY: Hospital Social Service Association of New York City. doi:https://play.google.com/store/books/details?id=j8UZAQAAIAAJ

Sydenstricker, E. (1928). The Decline in the Tuberculosis Death Rate in Cattaraugus County. *The Milbank Memorial Fund Quarterly Bulletin, 6*(2), 41-50. Doi: 10.2307/3347534

Szabo-Perricelli, C. (2016). *J. N. Adam Memorial Hospital: Her Inside Voice.* Buffalo, NY: People Ink Press in association with the Museum of disABILITY History

Supreme Court Appellate Division-Fourth Department. (1940). Walton, NY: The Reporter Company. doi: httsp://play.google.com/store/books/details?id=BZHxEfbbOQoC

Salvatore Messina against United States Gypsum Company

The New York Supplement. (1919). West Publishing Company. doi:https://play.google.com/store/books/details?id=3-IKAAAAYAAJ

The SUNY Buffalo Law School Clinical Legal Education Program. (2013). *A Neighborhood's Continuing Evolution* [Brochure]. Author. Retrieved February 9, 2019, from http://www.law.buffalo.edu/cle/130426/program-materials.html

Timeline. (2015, January 08). Retrieved January 15, 2018, from http://foodsystemhistory.wordpress.com/timeline/

Topics in Chronicling America - Pure Food and Drug Act of 1906. (n.d.). Retrieved February 02, 2019, from https://www.loc.gov/rr/news/topics/purefood.html

Treating Tuberculosis with Sunlight. (n.d.). Retrieved February 01, 2019, from http://www.weirduniverse.net/blog/comments/treating_tuberculosis_with_sunlight

Trends in Mortality of Tuberculosis Patients in the United ... (n.d.). Retrieved February 9, 2019, from https://www.ncbi.nlm.nih.gov/pmc/articles/PMC3166369/

Vaccines | Basic TB Facts | TB | CDC. (n.d.). Retrieved December 2, 2018, from https://www.cdc.gov/tb/topic/basics/vaccines.htm

Walsh, J. J. (1919). *History of Medicine in New York: Three Centuries of Medical Progression*(Vol. 3). National Americana Society. doi:https://play.google.com/store/books/details?id=fQsJAAAAIAAJ

PHOTOS

(1920) *Food and Tuberculosis.,* 1920. [New York: National Child Welfare Association: Co-operating with Natl. Assn. for the Study and Prevention of Tuberculosis, between ? and 1923?] [Photograph] Retrieved from the Library of Congress, https://www.loc.gov/item/2014647543/

(1920) *Open Air Schools and Tuberculosis,* 1920. [New York: National Child Welfare Association: Co-operating with Natl. Assn. for the Study and Prevention of Tuberculosis, between ? and 1923?] [Photograph] Retrieved from the Library of Congress, https://www.loc.gov/item/2014647548

(ca. 1890) *Leysin, the sanatorium and Chaussy in winter, Vaud, Canton of, Switzerland.,* ca. 1890. [Between and Ca. 1900] [Photograph] Retrieved from the Library of Congress, https://www.loc.gov/item/2001703352

Irma and Paul Milstein. Division of United States History, Local History and Genealogy, The New York Public Library. "Row of Outhouses" The New York Public Library Digital Collections. 1902-1904.

Ruslander, F. (1920). *The J.N.Adam Memorial Hospital: Perrysburg, New York.* Buffalo, NY: Russell Print. doi:http://resource.nlm.nih.gov/101242990